P9-EGN-643

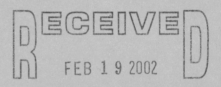

RECEIVED

FEB 1 9 2002

CASTRO VALLEY

NATURAL
HEALTH AT
50+

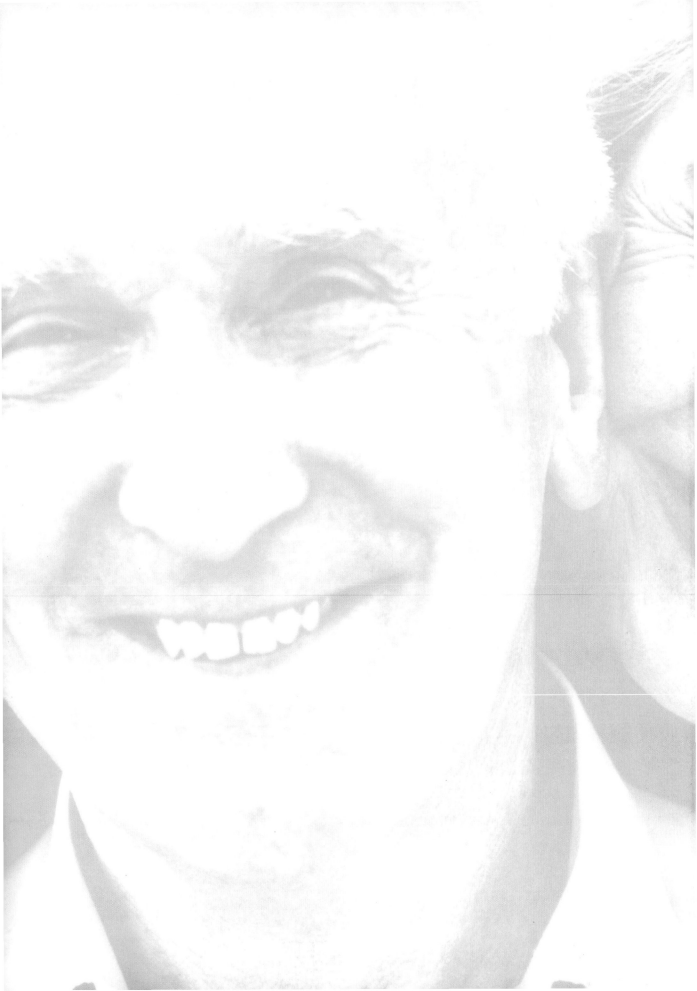

NATURAL
HEALTH AT
50+

The Vital Guide to Living Longer and Looking Good

Dr. Christina Scott-Moncrieff
MB ChB MFHom

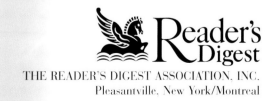

THE READER'S DIGEST ASSOCIATION, INC.
Pleasantville, New York/Montreal

A Reader's Digest Book

First published in Great Britain in 2001
by Collins & Brown Limited
London House
Great Eastern Wharf
Parkgate Road
London SW11 4NQ

Reader's Digest Project Staff
EDITORIAL DIRECTOR: Wayne Kalyn
SENIOR DESIGN DIRECTOR: Elizabeth L. Tunnicliffe
SENIOR DESIGNER: Carol Nehring
EDITORIAL MANAGER: Christine R. Guido

Reader's Digest Illustrated Reference Books
EDITOR-IN-CHIEF: Christopher Cavanaugh
ART DIRECTOR: Joan Mazzeo
DIRECTOR, TRADE PUBLISHING: Christopher T. Reggio
EDITORIAL DIRECTOR, TRADE: Susan Randol

1 3 5 7 9 8 6 4 2

Designed by Alison Lee, Creative Bubble
Edited by Claire Wedderburn-Maxwell, Connie Novis
Reproduction by Classic Scan Pte Ltd, Singapore
Printed and bound by C&C Offset, Hong Kong

Library of Congress Cataloging in Publication Data:
Scott-Moncrieff, Christina.
Natural health at 50+: the vital guide to living longer and looking good / Christina Scott-Moncrieff.
p. cm.
Includes bibliographical references and index.
ISBN 0-7621-0294-2
1. Longevity. 2. Health. 3. Physical fitness. 4. Aging – Prevention. I. Title: Natural health at fifty+. II. Title.

RA776.75 .S34 2001
613'.0434–dc21   00-042540

SAFETY NOTE
The information in this book is not intended as a substitute for medical advice.
Any person suffering from conditions requiring medical attention, or who has
symptoms that concern them, should consult a qualified medical practitioner.

CONTENTS

50 NOW: THE **WISDOM** YEARS

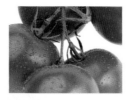

In developed countries today a healthy woman of 50 can expect to live another 30 years and a man another 26 years, but men should take heart as this gap is narrowing. Each year the number of people celebrating their hundredth birthday doubles, so for more and more people 50 is only the midpoint of their lives. To help you answer the challenge of making the most of the second half of your life, this book maps out an antiaging strategy that is designed to add "life to your years" as well as "years to your life."

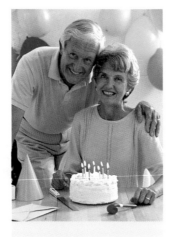

"Add life to your years as well as years to your life..."

In the first three decades of life, growing and maturing are much the same for most people. In the short term, whatever we throw at our bodies during these years, such as alcohol, tobacco smoke, and unhealthy eating habits, seems to make very little difference to our health. Then, at around 30+, there is a subtle change and maturing suddenly becomes reclassified as aging. Measures taken to combat the progress of aging cannot guarantee a long and healthy life, but they do increase the chances of longevity, and also of recovering good health rapidly if illness or an accident should unfortunately occur.

We all know how old we are in years. If you look around at your friends and relations of 50+, however, it is easy to see that some both look and move in ways that appear to be much older than their years. Others seem younger than 50+, and for them the biological clock seems to be moving more slowly. To some extent staying young is inherited, but scientists say that only about 30 percent of aging lies in the genes; the rest is up to you. So how can you slow the biological clock?

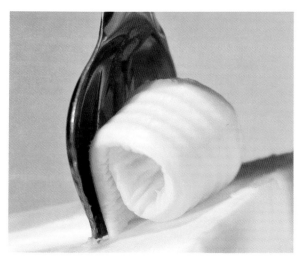

Oxygen reacts with other compounds to create free radicals. Its effects can be seen on butter left in a warm room, which degenerates into a rancid pool due to oxidation.

Biological aging

Doctors and scientists are gradually beginning to understand what causes aging, and this is the first step in devising ways to fight it. As we grow older the inner chemistry of our bodies becomes less efficient. Not only is it more likely to produce dangerous substances, known as free radicals, from internal chemical processes, but it is also less able to neutralize the free radicals that are produced as a result of external factors.

A free radical is a highly unstable molecule in which the electrical charge is unbalanced because one of the negatively charged electrons is missing. To restore electrical balance, the free radical grabs an electron from a nearby stable molecule, causing it to become a free radical. This sets up a chain reaction that can interfere with the normal activity of our cells, and eventually result in damage to our vital organs. Once the organs are damaged, the body is no longer able to function effectively, leaving the way open for chronic diseases to develop, perhaps 20 or 30 years later. However, this window of opportunity can be used to take measures that slow down these changes.

Surprisingly, oxygen is one of the most common generators of free radicals within the body. If you want to see the result of too much oxygen, leave a cube of butter, uncovered, in a warm kitchen. After a few days it degenerates into a yellow pool of fat that neither smells nor tastes like butter. Biologists believe that free radicals can cause similar serious damage to the fats that are contained in our brains and in the many cell membranes throughout our bodies. In butter the changes start fairly slowly because it contains substances, known as antioxidants, that neutralize free radicals, but once these antioxidants are used up the butter becomes rancid. Oxygen is, of course, essential to life, but its ability to produce free radicals can be controlled by eating plenty of antioxidants (see page 8).

If you eat food that is rancid you can increase the production of free radicals in your body. Rancidity can sometimes be tasted, as when wheat germ is no longer fresh it becomes bitter. More often there is no way to know how many free radicals you are eating. Oils, in particular, often undergo many chemical changes when they are exposed to light or heat. Shallow and deep-frying are the cooking methods that are most likely to produce free radicals and other harmful chemicals. These can build up in the body over the years causing long-term damage, even if fresh oil is used on each occasion. In commercial deep-frying, oils can be used at high temperatures for several consecutive days.

Another positive step is to try to minimize exposure to other sources of free radicals. These include:

■ Drugs, including tobacco smoke, marijuana smoke, alcohol, caffeine, and certain prescribed medications.

■ Toxic metals, such as lead from old paint and water pipes, cadmium from cigarette smoke, and the mercury present in certain industrial discharges.

■ Manufactured chemicals, many of which are difficult to detect, but come into your home, workplace, food, and water from many sources (see page 69).

■ Excessive exercise, causing your body to use oxygen more rapidly than when it is at rest, generates free radicals if you are short of

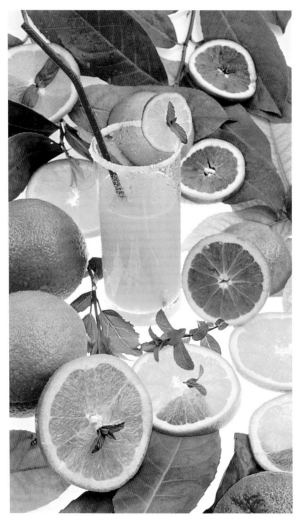

Eating generous amounts of fresh fruit and vegetables will provide you not only with a good source of vitamins, but also with vital antioxidants.

antioxidant vitamins and minerals in your diet (see below).

- Ionizing radiation, present in ultraviolet light, cosmic background radiation, and manmade sources, such as X rays.

Antioxidants in the diet

However hard we try it is obviously impossible to avoid all sources of free radicals, and our bodies have a number of well-developed defense systems that can neutralize them. Many of these systems rely on adequate supplies, in the diet, of substances known as antioxidants. These have the ability to halt the chain reactions that produce free radicals, and include beta carotene (or pro-vitamin A), vitamins C and E, and riboflavin, and the minerals copper, zinc, manganese, and selenium.

Of course, taking a handful of supplements may provide these antioxidants, but it is difficult to be sure that the balance is right. Supplements should only be taken to enhance a good diet, because they cannot provide the hundreds of carotenoids, bioflavonoids (see page 32), and other substances that are found in food and also have essential antioxidant functions. They are best obtained by eating generous amounts of a wide variety of fresh fruits and vegetables (see page 48).

Personalized antiaging

In addition to free radicals, stress is another cause of aging. To avoid the anxiety of making large and uncomfortable changes in your lifestyle you may find it helpful to develop your own antiaging plan. Lifestyle changes work best if they are introduced systematically over time. To be most beneficial they need to be prioritized and updated when more information becomes available or your circumstances change.

First of all, check out the risks you might have inherited. If diseases, such as heart disease, strokes, diabetes, cancer, or arthritis, have occurred frequently in your family this may indicate where you should start. Enlist your doctor's help and arrange for appropriate checkups. In

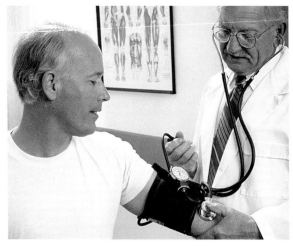

It is important to have your blood pressure checked regularly by your doctor.

any case having your blood pressure checked from time to time is strongly recommended at 50+, especially because many people who have high blood pressure aren't aware of it. High blood pressure can cause heart and kidney disease, and strokes.

Next look at those habits that can contribute to aging. Stop smoking (see page 70): five years after giving up you may have reduced your biological age by up to seven years. Reducing your alcohol intake to the recommended safe level (see page 71) can help de-age your mind and body. Regular exercise (see page 52) builds stamina and a healthier, stronger heart that may last several years longer if it is exercised. Even if you don't want to play sports or go to a gym, you can strengthen your heart and bones and simply feel younger by walking regularly. If you are over-weight do not try to lose the pounds all at once. However, a gradual weight loss (see pages 43 and 55) boosts morale and can both prolong life and improve your quality of life by reducing the risk of developing a number of illnesses, including arthritis, heart disease, diabetes, and some cancers.

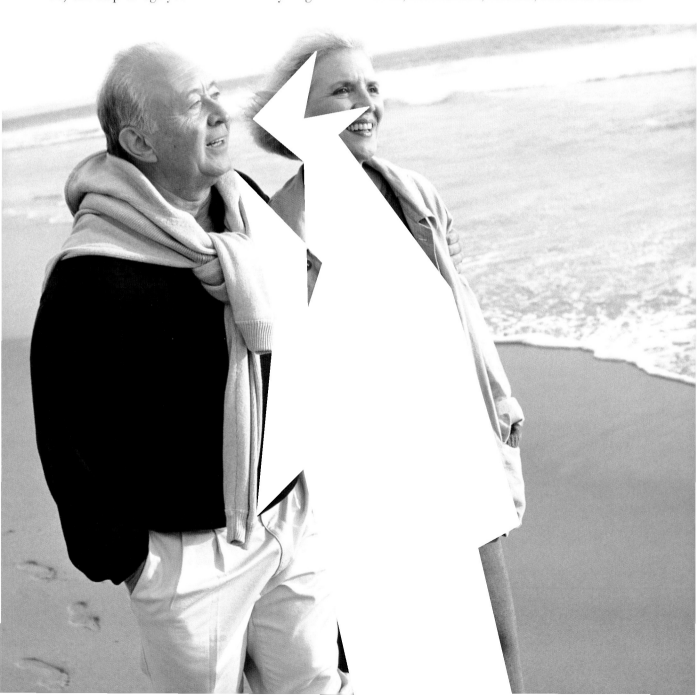

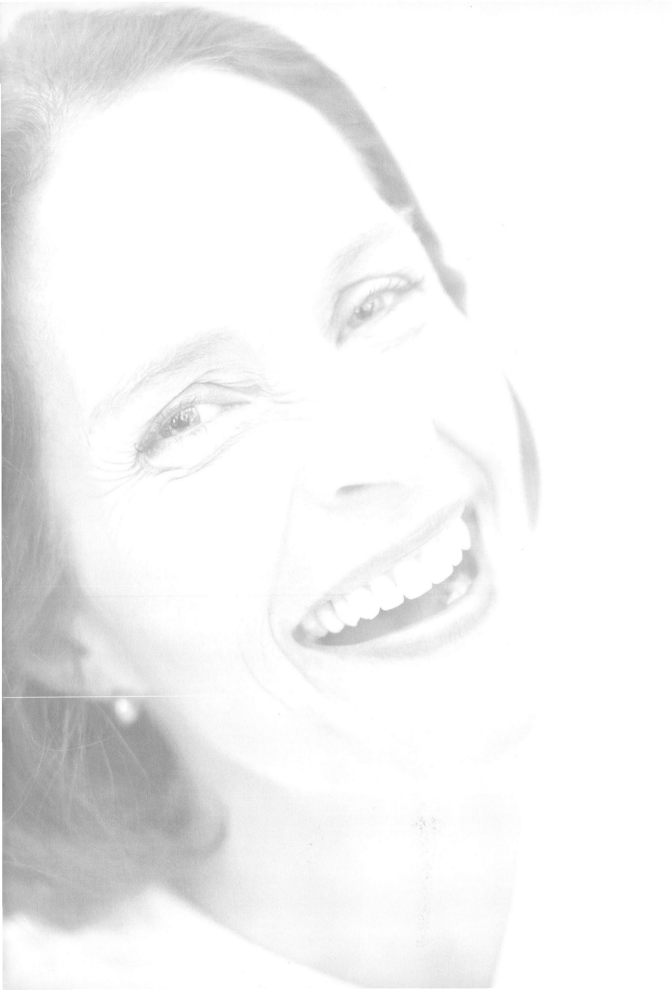

PART 1

LIVING FOR THE NEXT 50 YEARS

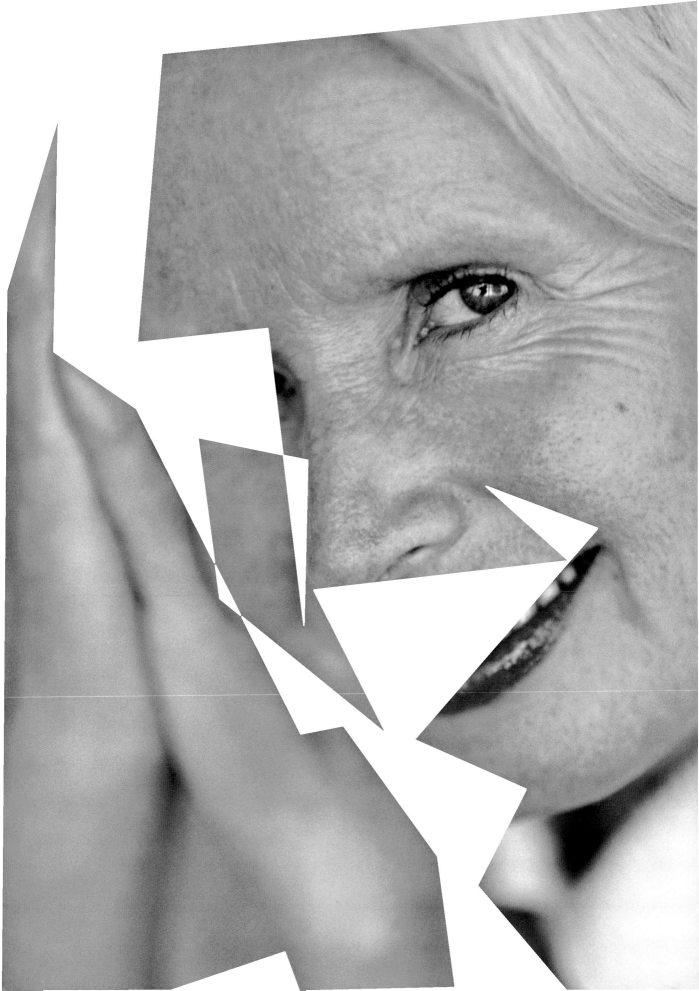

Chapter One

HEALTHY
EATING

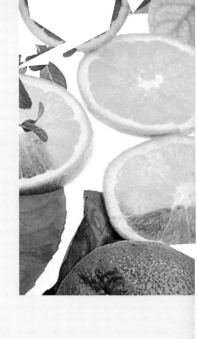

During the twentieth century scientific advances provided more information about the composition of the food we eat and expanded our knowledge of our nutritional needs. But science has also revealed how little we still know about the ways in which food affects our health. A welcome trend in recent years has been a willingness to examine the nutritional benefits of natural foods often eaten in less developed countries.

"Tell me what you eat and I will tell you what you are."

Anthelme Brillat-Savarin (1755–1826)

EATING FOR THE NEXT 50 YEARS

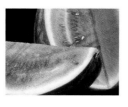

Many exciting developments are taking place in the science of nutrition. For example, scientists are beginning to understand why some people who live in less developed countries can survive into old age without being plagued by the degenerative diseases that occur in those living in so-called "developed" countries.

Old wives' tales, such as "eat your vegetables" or "an apple a day keeps the doctor away," are achieving scientific respectability as researchers discover that natural foods contain beneficial substances that can improve health (see Plant Power, page 32), and possibly fight off diseases such as cancer and heart disease. Even quite modest dietary changes can improve the quality of life within a few months.

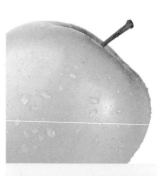

"An apple a day keeps the doctor away..."

It's not all in the genes

Everyone inherits a set of genes from each parent and that genetic legacy may predispose you to certain diseases. The more that doctors and nutritionists use nutritional means to treat people, the more they realize that just possessing a gene for a certain disease does not mean that an illness will inevitably develop. If the body is provided with a well-balanced and nutritious diet, it has the resources to discourage the faulty genes from expressing themselves. Your fiftieth birthday is a good time to consider the best dietary regime to adopt for the next 50 years, but even if you are much older, improving your diet can still achieve a surprising amount.

Our nutritional needs change throughout our lives. At 50+ we need fewer calories, but we still need the same quantity of minerals and vitamins, so the quality of our diet becomes more important.

Recommended energy intakes (calories/day)

	At 50	At 51+	
Men	2,900	2,300	These recommendations will not be enough if you are doing plenty of exercise or heavy physical work.
Women	2,200	1,900	

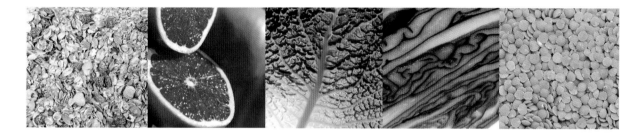

The Optimum Diet

A healthy diet contains plenty of unprocessed natural foods, such as fruit (2–4 portions each day), vegetables (3–5 portions each day), whole grains, beans, seeds, and nuts. Nonvegetarians can add modest amounts of lean meat and fish. Such a diet provides a good supply of the four major food groups:

■ Carbohydrates for energy (see page 16).

■ Protein to repair the body tissues and immune system and maintain a healthy brain (see page 18).

■ Fats for energy reserves, and many other functions (see page 19), including maintaining a healthy nervous system and brain.

■ Fiber for a healthy digestive system and to reduce the risk of heart disease (see page 22).

■ Water is also essential for concentration, energizing the body, and decreasing the risk of kidney stones and gallstones (see page 23).

Vitamins and minerals

Vitamins and minerals are only needed in small amounts, but they are essential for health. How much of these minor nutrients we need has been

very difficult to calculate because individuals have different needs, and the amounts that are contained in any given food can vary enormously. For example, some supermarket oranges have been found to contain no vitamin C.

Historically, government organizations have made specific recommendations for the minimum daily intake of certain vitamins and minerals by basing their calculations on the avoidance of disease (see pages 27–31). Most nutritionists, however, now believe that it would be preferable to base the minimum daily intake on the amount needed to achieve health. This is even more difficult to measure, however, because "health" is not easily defined.

Taking supplements

At 50+, obtaining sufficient vitamins and minerals is more necessary than ever for those who want to stay looking and feeling good, and to reduce the risks of becoming ill. Many people take supplements, but these must be regarded as *supplementary* to a diet that is as healthy as it can be made, and not as an *alternative* to eating well. This is because natural foods contain a huge number of different substances (see Plant Power, page 32) that are only being identified now. It will be many years before their functions are fully understood, and eating the Optimum Diet means that you will be obtaining them naturally every day.

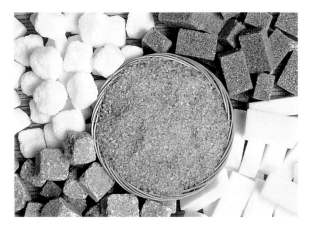

Refined sugar should be eaten as a treat, rather than as an everyday food.

Carbohydrate

Carbohydrate foods consist of sugar molecules, which have a number of chemical arrangements. As a result, they are digested and absorbed in different ways. Single sugar molecules are glucose and fructose (fruit sugar), double molecules are sucrose (the "sugar" in your bowl), maltose (in germinating grain), and lactose (in milk). Starches are made up of long chains of sugar molecules, usually glucose. As a result they take longer to be digested and absorbed, so the sugar is released slowly and its level in the blood remains steady. Apart from fructose, which is released from fruit relatively slowly, foods that contain single and double sugar molecules are usually absorbed more quickly than starchy foods.

These different rates of absorption are important. If your intake of rapidly absorbed sugars is high, the level of glucose in your blood will go up too quickly, even though this is only temporary if your pancreas is working well and producing sufficient insulin to remove the sugar from the bloodstream. The raised glucose increases the likelihood that some of it will become attached to protein molecules, producing "advanced glycation end products," or A.G.Es. It is likely that these may contribute to some of the changes of aging, including arthritis, cataracts, and heart disease, all of which occur earlier in people with diabetes in whom raised blood sugar levels are common. In addition, energy levels and sugar cravings are easier to control when you eat starchy foods because your body releases the sugar they contain

gradually. Sugars that have been refined by food manufacturers, such as those found in cakes, cookies, candies, and chocolate, should be eaten as occasional treats rather than as a regular part of the diet.

How much carbohydrate is best?

Between 55 and 70 percent of the Optimum Diet should come from carbohydrate-rich foods. This means that, over a day, around two thirds of the food you eat should consist of fruit, vegetables, and wholegrain foods.

Ideally, about 80 percent of carbohydrate should come from foods that release their sugar slowly, such as vegetables, including raw root vegetables, legumes, and certain fresh fruits (see box). These also contain plenty of water or, as in legumes, a proportion of protein. As a result the carbohydrate they contain is less dense, so you can eat plenty of them, to ensure that you obtain a good supply of vitamins and minerals, without putting on weight or causing blood sugar levels to rise too rapidly. The remaining 20 percent should come from foods that contain more densely packed carbohydrates, such as whole grains, cooked starchy vegetables, and dried fruits, or from fruits that have been shown to release sugar more rapidly, such as bananas, oranges, melons, mangoes, and pineapples. These foods contain valuable minerals and vitamins too, and should not be avoided altogether.

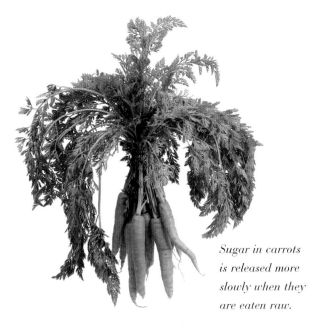

Sugar in carrots is released more slowly when they are eaten raw.

As far as possible try to eat carbohydrate food that is close to its natural state. Grains, and foods made from grains, should be unrefined, such as wholewheat flour and bread, and brown pasta and rice. These are more filling and nutritious than products made from white flour and sugar, which have had many nutrients removed during the refining processes. Eat the skins of potatoes and fruit to increase your intake of fiber (see page 22). Fiber in foods slows down the rate of digestion, preventing a peak in blood sugar levels and insulin. Have whole fresh fruit instead of fruit juice, because the juice releases sugar more quickly and contains less fiber.

Sugars from these foods are absorbed gradually

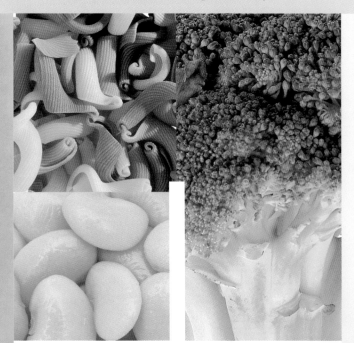

Grains

Pearl barley, oatmeal, buckwheat, pasta

Legumes

All beans, peas, lentils, peanuts, garbanzo beans, flour, soy milk

Vegetables

All, except cooked starchy or root vegetables, such as beets, carrots, parsnips, pumpkins, corn, potatoes, sweet potatoes

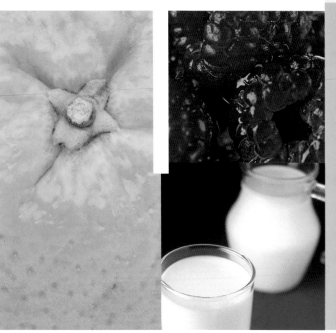

Fruit

Apples, apricots, fresh pears, grapes, cherries, plums, grapefruit

Fruit sugar

Fructose

Dairy products

Low-fat milk, yogurt (without added sugar)

Protein

Protein is made up of base units known as amino acids. Amino acids are the only dietary source of nitrogen, which is needed to maintain and repair the protein structures in the body, such as muscles, hormones, and parts of the immune system. In human beings, proteins are made from 21 amino acids, of which about eight are described as "essential" for adults. This means they have to be eaten in the diet. Provided the total intake of protein is adequate, all the other amino acids can be made in the body.

During digestion, proteins are broken down into amino acids. These amino acids are used to construct new proteins used by the immune system, or to make hormones or the enzymes needed to facilitate many of the chemical changes in the body, including digestion. Very little protein is stored, so it should be eaten every day, and preferably as part of every meal.

Where are proteins found?

For most people the main sources of protein are meat, fish, eggs, milk, and milk products, but even nonvegetarians obtain up to half their protein from vegetable and grain sources (such as whole grains), beans, nuts, and seeds. Even fruit and vegetables contain very small amounts of protein. Until recently, it was thought the source of protein did not matter, but it is now believed that the way that the body uses animal protein differs from its use of vegetable protein. An excessive amount of protein from animal sources may increase the risk of developing a number of diseases, including high blood pressure, certain cancers, and osteoporosis.

How much protein is required?

Despite extensive research, the exact amount of protein needed for optimum health is not known for certain. Some scientific studies suggest that older people need more than younger people, while others suggest the opposite. An additional complication is that much of the research has been directed toward avoiding protein deficiency, rather than finding the optimum intake.

At present, the recommended daily intake of protein at 50+ is 0.8mg for each kilogram (or 2.2 pounds) of body weight. This works out at about 2oz (around 56g) for a person of average weight. Current recommendations suggest that we should not eat more than double the recommended intake of protein. (See page 49 if you do not eat protein from animal sources.)

A guide to protein in food

Each of these portions contains about 12g (just under half an ounce) of protein:

2oz (60g) lean meat
2oz (60g) fish
1½oz (45g) cheddar cheese
14oz (400ml) skim milk
3½oz (100g) oatmeal (uncooked)
3½oz (100g) puffed wheat
4½oz (130g) wholewheat bread
2oz (60g) peanuts
3½oz (100g) walnuts
2oz (60g) sunflower seeds
5oz (150g) tofu
6oz (170g) red kidney beans (cooked)

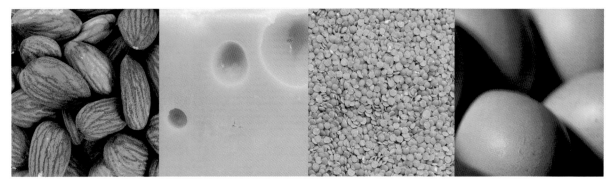

Protein is needed for the repair of body tissues, and is best obtained from a variety of food sources.

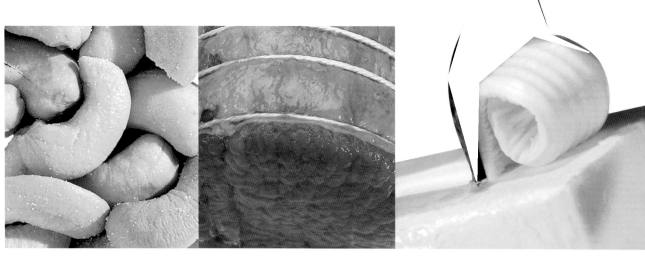

The fat in nuts, such as cashews, is richer in healthy monounsaturated fat than the fat found in red meat and whole dairy products, which is mostly of the saturated variety.

Fat

Fat is an important component of the diet: it is present in every cell membrane and is essential for the nervous system to function normally. Fat is also needed to enable fat-soluble vitamins (see page 24) to be absorbed from the diet and used by the body's cells. A major problem with fat is that it contains twice as many calories as either protein or carbohydrate. Any fat that is not burned to release energy is stored in the body as fatty tissue, but it can also be deposited in major arteries. To avoid obesity and reduce the risk of developing heart disease and some cancers, it is best to limit your fat intake to 25–30 percent of calories: this is 55–66g daily if you eat a 2,000-calorie-a-day diet. This is less fat than the average eaten by most people in developed countries, but more than in some of the very low-fat diets that have been promoted in recent years.

Fat consists of long chains of carbon atoms surrounded by variable numbers of hydrogen atoms. Fats that are solid at room temperature are called saturated fats, because all the chemical bonds are filled, or "saturated," by hydrogen. In general, these fats should be eaten sparingly because, when eaten in excess, they have been linked with heart disease, strokes, obesity, multiple sclerosis, and cancer. Saturated fats are found in red meat, full-fat dairy products such as whole milk, butter, and cheese, and certain plants, such as coconut. People with heart disease are often advised to avoid them altogether.

Unsaturated fats are usually soft at room temperature and we recognize them as oils. These fats are "unsaturated" because some of the chemical bonds are unfilled. Unsaturated fats are sometimes called "good" fats, and they should provide 65–80 percent of the fat you eat. There are two types: mono- and polyunsaturated fats. Monounsaturated fat is found in olives, almonds, avocados, peanuts, pecans, cashews, hazelnuts, and macadamia nuts, and it appears to provide some protection against heart disease. Because they have only one unfilled bond in each molecule, these oils may become solid in cold weather or in a refrigerator, but this is not harmful.

Polyunsaturated fats have at least two unfilled bonds, which means that they are chemically less stable and more likely to be affected by light, heat, oxygen, and the presence of other chemicals. This can be a problem when they are hydrogenated into "trans fats": these are fats that the body cannot easily use and are likely to cause blockage of the arteries. Trans fats are often contained in margarine and snack foods.

The best sources of unsaturated fats are natural cold-pressed oils, whole seeds and nuts, oily fruit, such as avocados, and oily fish. Olive oil and canola oil are best to cook with because they are more stable when heated than corn, safflower, and soybean oils.

Essential fats

Some polyunsaturated fats are known as "essential fats" because they cannot be made in our bodies and have to come from the diet. They are present in all whole, unprocessed foods, including dark green vegetables, leaves, and herbs, such as spinach, parsley, and broccoli.

There are two types of essential fat: linoleic from the omega-6 family of fats, and linolenic from the omega-3 family. Today, you are relatively unlikely to eat a diet that is deficient in omega-6 fats, but this is not true of the omega-3 fats. Dr. Udo Erasmus, a biochemist from Vancouver, Canada, has studied fats in the diet and believes that we are now eating only one sixth of the omega-3 oils that were found in the food supply in the mid-1800s. Because they become rancid easily, omega-3 oils are removed during food processing to extend the shelf life of the foods that naturally contain them. In addition, the fat from modern farm-reared animals contains less omega-3 fat than that from wild animals.

Even though we need less omega-3 oil than omega-6, Dr. Erasmus and a number of other scientists now believe that we are eating disproportionately too much omega-6 fat.

What essential fats do

If your diet contains very little fat you may not be obtaining enough essential fats. These help to:

- Maintain energy levels and combat fatigue.

- Prevent food cravings and maintain steady levels of sugar in the blood.

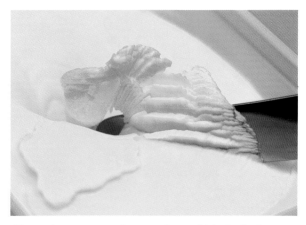

Margarine may contain trans fats, which the body cannot easily use, and which contribute to heart disease. Soft margarines are best as they contain fewer trans fats.

- Reduce depression.

- Bolster your immune system.

- Keep your skin soft and youthful.

- Possibly reduce the risk of developing cancer.

Making "better butter"

Margarine is not necessarily preferable to butter because it often contains trans fats (see above). The truth is that we should be eating less of both, but you can reduce the saturated fat content of butter if you blend equal weights of butter with either olive oil or canola oil.

Unlike some margarine, this mixture contains very few trans fats, but is soft even when it is refrigerated. It is still, however, fat and should be used sparingly.

Rich sources of essential fats

Omega-3 fats	Omega-6 fats	Foods that contain both
Oily fish	Safflower oil	Soybeans
Flaxseed (linseed) oil	Sunflower oil	Walnuts
	Sesame seed oil	

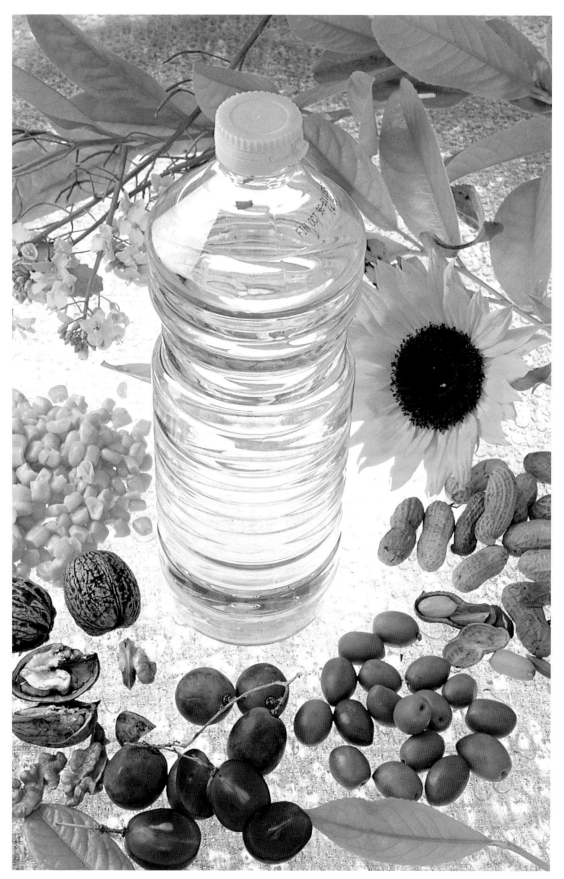

Sunflower oil is a good source of omega-6 fats, but these need to be balanced with sufficient omega-3 fats.

Guide to the fiber content of foods

Food	Grams of fiber per 3¹/₂oz (100g)
Fruits	2–4
Berries	7–9
Cooked beans	5–7
Vegetables	1–2
Wholegrain bread	7.5
Beans	4–7

Fiber

Fiber is the indigestible parts of plants. Insufficient fiber in the diet is linked to many diseases, including heart disease, gallstones, diabetes, arthritis, certain cancers, diseases of the colon, and obesity.

Dietary fiber is best obtained from foods that are as near to their natural state as possible, such as brown rice, wholewheat bread and wholegrain cereal, whole fruit including the skin, and vegetables, especially legumes. Nuts and seeds also contain plenty of fiber. They are high in calories, however, and should be eaten only in small amounts even though the fat they contain is rich in essential fats (see page 20). It is best to obtain fiber from whole foods and avoid supplements such as wheat bran, which in large amounts can limit absorption of vital minerals such as calcium, iron, and zinc.

Natural unrefined foods provide two forms of fiber that have been shown to reduce the risk of developing a number of diseases.

How does fiber help?

Fiber assists in controlling appetite by ensuring that you feel full for longer after a meal, and at the same time it regulates the release of glucose into the bloodstream (see pages 16–17). Insoluble fiber, found in whole wheat, corn, and brown rice, increases the bulk of the stool, reducing the risk of both constipation and the development of diverticular disease, in which the wall of the colon (large bowel) is weakened, and helps to prevent hemorrhoids (piles). Soluble fiber, which occurs in apples, carrots, barley, and oats, helps to reduce cholesterol and to balance sugar levels in the blood.

How much fiber is needed?

In North America the average intake of fiber for adults has been calculated to be about 12g a day (just under ½ oz). The Food and Nutrition Board recommend that this should be increased to 25–35g through increased consumption of fruit, vegetables, and wholegrain products.

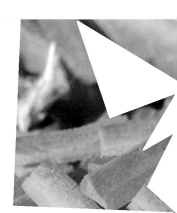

Water

Drinking sufficient water is essential for health, yet as many as half of all North Americans are mildly dehydrated. Almost two thirds of the human body consists of water. We can do without food for much longer than we can survive without water, but we do need a supply as free of pollutants and chemicals as we can get. You can purchase high-quality water filters that remove pollutants, but not minerals. The cartridges in water filters should be replaced regularly to prevent harmful microbes from collecting inside. It is best not to use filters that remove calcium and magnesium from hard water because these minerals appear to reduce the risk of heart attacks and strokes.

Water is lost from the body through the kidneys, skin, and lungs. Physiologists calculate that adults need to produce at least 2 cups (half a liter) of urine each day to remove waste products. In addition, even on a cool day, a minimum of 4 cups (1 liter) of water is lost through the lungs and skin – more when you are sweating.

To be on the safe side, an intake of water that is double the minimum loss is needed. Much, if not all, of this safety margin can be obtained by eating about seven portions of fruit and vegetables each day. So adults eating the Optimum Diet need to drink *at least* an additional 4–6 cups (1–1½ liters) of water each day, and more in hot weather, or when exercising strenuously. Don't rely on thirst to tell you when to drink more, though; as we age, thirst becomes a less sensitive indication of dehydration. Large amounts of tea, coffee, and alcoholic drinks are not recommended because they act on the kidneys to increase the amount of urine that is produced, and increase the amount of other substances, such as caffeine and alcohol, that have to be processed and removed from the body.

Water power

Drinking enough liquid can:

■ Increase concentration.

■ Energize your body.

■ Maximize your immune system.

■ Help prevent constipation.

■ Rehydrate the skin.

■ Lower the risk of developing gallstones, kidney stones, and even bladder cancer.

VITAMINS

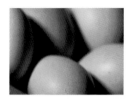

There are two categories of vitamins: those that are soluble in water and those that are soluble in fat. Because the water-soluble vitamins can be excreted in the urine, they are not particularly toxic, except at very high doses. Apart from vitamin B_{12}, which is stored in the liver, try to eat foods that contain water-soluble vitamins every day. If you wish to take supplements, the B vitamins work together and need to be balanced. It is best to seek professional advice if you want to take supplements of single B vitamins. Or, choose an over-the-counter multivitamin because the manufacturer usually balances doses of individual B vitamins.

Fat-soluble vitamins (vitamins A, D, E, and K) are toxic at lower doses than water-soluble vitamins, but they are also stored for longer in the body and do not have to be taken every day. If you wish to take supplements, it is best to take fat-soluble vitamins in only one preparation at any one time, and to follow the manufacturer's instructions carefully so that you do not take too much.

Vitamin A: Retinol and beta-carotene
Needed for: good vision, especially at night; healthy skin and mucous membranes; a healthy immune system.
Good sources: fortified milk, eggs, liver, butter, enriched margarine, and fish liver oils. All of these contain preformed vitamin A (retinol). In addition, vitamin A is made in the body, from beta-carotene, found in red and yellow vegetables and fruit, such as sweet potatoes, spinach, bell peppers, carrots, tomatoes, and apricots.
Cautions: toxic when eaten or supplemented in

large amounts as vitamin A. Do not exceed 4,000 IU a day for women and 5,000 IU a day for men. There are no known toxic side effects from beta-carotene.

Vitamin B_1: Thiamin
Needed for: maintaining energy levels; a healthy nervous system.
Good sources: lean pork, whole grains, fortified breakfast cereals, legumes, nuts, and seeds.
Can be lost: when food is boiled or steamed. Absorption in the intestine is reduced when alcohol is also present.
Cautions: can be toxic in high doses.

Vitamin B_2: Riboflavin
Needed for: good vision; healthy hair, skin, and nails; maintaining energy levels; combating stress.
Good sources: milk, cheese, yogurt, eggs, beef, fish, mushrooms, and fortified breakfast cereals.

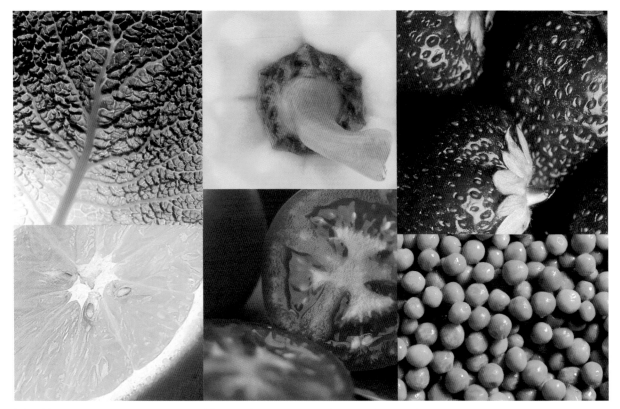

A healthy diet contains 2–4 portions of fruit and 3–5 portions of vegetables each day.

Can be lost: when the food containing riboflavin is exposed to light. Such foods should be stored in the dark.

Vitamin B₃: Niacin, Niacinamide, Nicotinic acid, Nicotinositol hexaniacinate

Needed for: energy; brain function; healthy skin; controlling cholesterol levels.

Good sources: beef, pork, chicken, white fish, wholewheat bread, eggs, baked beans, peas, and fortified breakfast cereals.

Can be lost: up to 90 percent is removed when whole grains are milled.

Cautions: can cause blood pressure to fall. Consult your doctor before taking supplements if you have any medical condition.

Vitamin B₅: Pantothenic acid

Needed for: the release of energy from food.

Good sources: legumes, meat, eggs, fish, wheat germ, and many other foods. Dietary deficiency has not been reported.

Can be lost: during cooking and from grains during milling.

Vitamin B₆: Pyridoxine

Needed for: new red blood cells; a healthy immune system.

Good sources: meat, fish, poultry, eggs, whole cereals, peas, avocados, and bananas.

Can be lost: when food is exposed to sunlight, during cooking, milling of grains.

Cautions: can be toxic in high doses.

Vitamin B₁₂: Cyanocobalamin

Needed for: new blood cells; protection of nerve cells; to enable all cells to function efficiently.

Good sources: milk, cheese, eggs, meat, fish, fortified breakfast cereals, and brewer's yeast.

Folic acid or Folate

Needed for: red blood cell production; healthy skin, hair, and nerves.

Good sources: green leafy vegetables, organ meats, brewer's yeast, and fortified breakfast cereals.

Can be lost: when food is exposed to light and heat (even room temperature).

Cautions: can be toxic in high doses. Consult your doctor before taking supplements if you take medication for epilepsy or have a family history of pernicious anemia.

Biotin

Needed for: healthy skin and nails; the absorption of vitamin C.

Good sources: fruit, nuts, sardines, and eggs. Ample amounts are normally made in the intestine.

Vitamin C: Ascorbate, Ascorbic acid

Needed for: healthy connective tissue and immune system.

Good sources: kiwi fruits, mangoes, citrus fruits, bell peppers, tomatoes, potatoes, cauliflowers, and cabbage.

Can be lost: during cooking.

Cautions: reduce the dose if you develop diarrhea when taking a supplement. Also, consult your doctor before taking supplements if you or a relative have had kidney stones.

Vitamin D

Needed for: healthy bones; balancing minerals in the body.

Good sources: herring, kippers, salmon, sardines, fortified margarine and breakfast cereals, and cod and halibut liver oils. Vitamin D is added to milk; one cup contains 100 IU.

Cautions: toxic in large amounts, although the threshold for toxicity is unknown. Consult your doctor before taking a supplement if you have sarcoidosis.

Vitamin E: Tocopherol

Needed for: neutralizing free radicals (see page 7); protecting the fats in cell membranes.

Good sources: vegetable oils, nuts, seeds, and wheat germ.

Can be lost: during food processing, such as milling, cooking, and freezing; or when food is stored, especially if exposed to the air – for example, unshelled nuts.

Although vitamins and minerals are only needed in small quantities, they are essential for health.

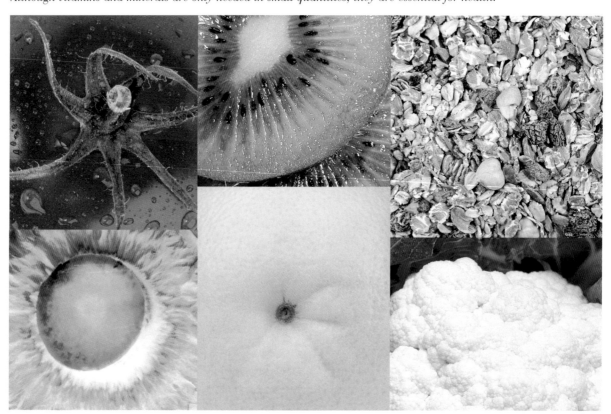

Cautions: consult your doctor before taking a supplement if you have high blood pressure or take anticoagulant medication.

Vitamin K: Phylloquinone, Menadione

Needed for: blood clotting, helping to build strong bones.

Good sources: many vegetables, including spinach, cabbage, cauliflower, and peas.

Cautions: consult your doctor before taking a supplement if you take anticoagulant medication. Synthetic vitamin K (Menadione) can be toxic and if a supplement is taken do not exceed the recommended daily intake (see below).

Vitamins: recommendations for minimum daily intake at 50+

Fat-soluble vitamins

Vitamin	RDA (US)		RNI (Can)	
	Male	Female	Male	Female
A	5,000IU	4,000IU	1,000mcg	800mcg
D	400–600IU	400–600IU	2.5mcg	2.5mcg
E	33IU	22IU	9.0mg	6.0mg
K (mcg)	80	65	80*	65*

Water-soluble vitamins

Vitamin	RDA (US)		RNI (Can)	
	Male	Female	Male	Female
B_1 (mg)	1.2	1.1	1.1	0.8
B_2 (mg)	1.3	1.1	1.4	1
B_3 (mg)	16	14	19	14
B_5 (mg)	4–7*	4–7*	4–7*	4–7*
B_6 (mg)	2.0	1.6	2.0*	1.6*
B_{12} (mcg)	2.4	2.4	1.0	1.0
Biotin (mcg)	30–100*	30–100*	30–100*	30–100*
C (mg)	60	60	40	40
Folate (mcg)	400	400	230	185

Notes

* These are the estimated safe and adequate daily dietary intake. Recommended daily allowances (US)/recommended nutrient intake (Canada) has not been established; values are based on current expert opinions.

mcg = microgram; mg = milligram; IU = International unit.

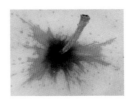

MINERALS

Minerals are chemical elements that are obtained from the Earth's crust. They are needed in the structures of the body or for the many biochemical processes that sustain life. Minerals can be grouped in two categories: the major minerals and the microminerals.

Unlike some of the vitamins, minerals cannot be made in the body and have to be gained from the diet. There is some concern that mineral deficiencies may be more common than vitamin deficiencies partly because many of the minerals, normally absorbed by plants from the soil, have not been replaced when chemical fertilizers are applied.

In addition, the distribution of minerals in the Earth's crust is variable, so the soil in some areas can be naturally low in essential minerals.

Certain processes within the food industry remove vital minerals from natural foods. For example, all the minerals and vitamins in sugar beet or sugar cane are lost when these are processed to yield refined white sugar. Fortunately, blackstrap molasses, which is a by-product of sugar refining, can be a useful and nutritious sweetener. When wheat is milled to white flour, more than 80 percent of the zinc, chromium, magnesium, and manganese are lost – all of which are essential for health.

The Major Minerals

These are the minerals that are found in the greatest amounts in the body, and a number of them contribute to the infrastructure of the body, such as calcium in the bones.

Calcium, magnesium, and phosphorus

These three minerals act together to maintain healthy bones, relay messages along nerves, and enable muscles to function normally. However, they compete with one another for absorption in the intestine.

Phosphorus is the most easily absorbed, and can be disproportionately high in a diet that contains too much animal protein or carbonated drinks, such as sodas. Hard water can supply useful amounts of both calcium and magnesium.

Calcium

Additional functions: enables blood to clot; may help to prevent colon cancer and lower blood pressure.

Good sources: milk and milk products, canned

sardines including the bones, beans, and green leafy vegetables.

Cautions: a high intake of calcium, when magnesium intake is inadequate, can cause kidney stones. It can also be deposited in soft tissue, such as in muscle and the walls of arteries.

Magnesium

Additional functions: helps to release energy from food; enables muscles to relax, including the muscles of arteries, which may help to control blood pressure.

Good sources: legumes, nuts, dark green vegetables, shellfish, wholewheat bread, blackstrap molasses, walnuts, and bananas.

Phosphorus

Additional functions: vital for energy production; helps certain B vitamins to function effectively.

Good sources: cheese, eggs, wholewheat bread, meat, peanuts, shrimp, walnuts, and yogurt.

Cautions: excessive phosphorus may be one cause of calcium deficiency and possibly of osteoporosis.

Sodium, potassium, and chloride

The balance between these three minerals is vital in regulating the amount of water in the body and the delicate balance of its distribution in the tissues and inside the cells. In general, the Western diet contains too much added salt, which consists of sodium and chloride, and this can lead to fluid imbalance. The exchange of sodium and potassium across the walls of cells enables muscles to relax and contract, and messages to be sent along nerve fibers.

Sodium

Good sources: bacon, ham, salted or smoked fish, olives in brine, pretzels, and bread.

(Note: when a food label specifies salt, you can calculate the sodium content by dividing the figure given for the amount of salt by 2.5.)

Potassium

Additional functions: helps to avoid fatigue and depression; helps to regulate blood pressure.

Good sources: all fruit and vegetables, nuts,

At 50+, feeling good will take a little more work than at 25, but it is well worth the effort.

pumpkin seeds, meat, and molasses. Salt substitute contains potassium chloride.

Chloride
Additional functions: essential for the hydrochloric acid secreted by the stomach for digestion.
Good sources: food to which salt or salt substitute has been added, such as tomato juice, and celery.

Silicon
Needed for: strong but supple, bones, arteries, cartilage, and tendons; may help prevent osteoporosis, osteoarthritis, high blood pressure, and Alzheimer's disease.
Good sources: hard water, unrefined grains, root vegetables, onions, and alfalfa sprouts.

Sulfur
Needed for: healthy skin, hair, nails, and immune system.
Good sources: protein foods, especially egg yolks, garlic, onions, and vegetables of the brassica family, such as broccoli, cabbage, and Brussels sprouts.

The Microminerals

These minerals are found in small amounts in the body. Many of them are an essential part of one or more enzymes, which are proteins that act as catalysts for the normal biochemical activity of the body.

Boron
Needed for: healthy bones; normal brain function.
Good sources: noncitrus fruit, leafy vegetables, nuts, and legumes.

Chromium
Needed for: stabilizing blood sugar levels, lowering cholesterol, and maintaining optimum body weight.
Good sources: brewer's yeast, molasses, whole grains, and vegetables.

Copper
Needed for: production of blood cells, and as part of the body's protection against free radicals.

Good sources: shellfish, liver, brewer's yeast, olives, wholewheat flour, walnuts, peanuts, and avocados.
Cautions: high doses can depress zinc levels; can be toxic in high doses.

Iodine
Needed for: thyroid hormones, which regulate energy production.
Good sources: fish, seaweed such as kelp, sea salt, milk, and eggs when iodine is fed to farm animals.

Iron
Needed for: distributing oxygen to all parts of the body in the blood.
Good sources: red meat, liver, wholewheat bread, fortified breakfast cereals, soy sauce, watercress, and green vegetables. Absorbed best when foods containing vitamin C are eaten at the same time.
Cautions: men and postmenopausal women should take iron supplements with caution. It can accumulate in the tissues and may predispose them to heart disease.

Manganese
Needed for: healthy bones and cartilage.
Good sources: whole grains, nuts, meat, dairy products, black tea, and ginger.

Molybdenum
Needed for: its contribution to the body's protection against free radicals.
Good sources: milk and milk products, legumes, organ meats (liver and kidney).

Selenium
Needed for: its powerful antioxidant function.
Good sources: Brazil nuts, shellfish, molasses, eggs, milk, and whole grains.
Cautions: can be toxic in high doses.

Zinc
Needed for: healthy immune system; normal sexual function in men.
Good sources: meat, eggs, fish, wholewheat bread, Brazil nuts, sesame seeds, and brewer's yeast.
Cautions: high doses can depress copper levels; can be toxic in high doses.

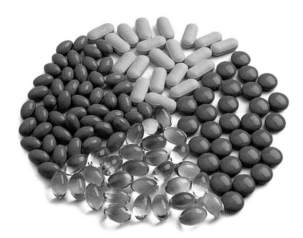

Taking mineral and vitamin supplements should be regarded as a health insurance policy to complement a healthy diet.

Minerals: recommendations for minimum daily intake at 50+

	RDA (US) Male	Female	RNI (Can) Male	Female
Boron (mg)	1*	1*	1*	1*
Calcium (mg)	1,000–1,200	1,000–1,200	800	1000–1500[1]
Chromium	50–200*mcg	50–200*mcg	0.05–0.2mg*	0.05–0.2mg*
Copper (mg)	1.5-3	1.5-3	2–3*	2–3*
Iodine (mcg)	150	150	160	160
Iron (mg)	10	15	9	9–13
Magnesium (mg)	350	280	250	200
Manganese (mg)	2–5*	2–5*	2–5*	2–5*
Molybdenum (mcg)	150–500*	150–500*	150–500*	150–500*
Phosphorus (mg)	700	700	1,000	850
Potassium	2,000*mg	2,000*mg	2–6g	2–6g
Selenium (mcg)	70	55	70	55
Silicon (mg)	5–10*	5–10*	5–10*	5–10*
Sodium	1,100–3,000*mg	1,100–3,000*mg	1–3g*	1–3g*
Zinc (mg)	15	12	12	9

Notes:

* These are the estimated safe and adequate daily dietary intake. Recommended daily allowances (US)/recommended nutrient intake (Canada) has not been established; values are based on current expert opinions.

[1] Post-menopause. 800mg before menopause.

mcg = microgram; mg = milligram; IU = International unit.

PLANT POWER

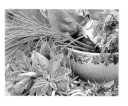

The Mediterranean diet has been praised as one of the healthiest in the world. It is a good example of the Optimum Diet (see page 15) with its generous provision of brightly colored vegetables, small portions of animal and fish protein, and the use of monounsaturated olive oil. One of the great secrets of the Mediterranean diet is the phytochemicals that are contained in brightly colored fresh produce.

Plants produce phytochemicals to protect themselves against natural hazards. When eaten by people and animals, this protection is passed on. Phytochemicals are particularly important for their antioxidant power, which helps to neutralize dangerous free radicals. More free radicals are produced at 50+ than during earlier years, and phytochemicals may reduce the risk of their causing illnesses, such as cancer, arthritis, and heart disease, among others.

Carotenoids

Carotenoids are some of the green, red, and yellow pigments that protect plants from too much sunlight. At one time, the main interest in carotenoids was the body's ability to convert beta-carotene into vitamin A. More recently, however, scientists have become interested in the antioxidant role performed by many other carotenoids. These are being shown to reduce the risk of cancer along with a wide range of diseases that are most common in older people.

Supplements

At present, the best advice is to obtain your carotenoids from fruits and vegetables because there is increasing scientific evidence for their health benefits. Experiments using supplements have yielded mixed results, and there is some concern that synthetic forms of beta-carotene may not be as effective as natural beta-carotene. It is also possible that getting a wide range of carotenoids is more effective than focusing on just one.

Flavonoids

These are plant pigments of many colors with powerful antioxidant activity. They help to damp down allergic conditions, such as asthma and hay fever, and inflammatory conditions, such as rheumatoid arthritis. They provide protection against viruses and carcinogens.

The citrus bioflavonoids and the proanthocyani-dins (PCOs; see box) strengthen the blood capillaries and improve the flow of blood inside them. This minimizes bleeding and bruising after an injury, and reduces symptoms such as tired, restless legs at the end of the day, and cramps at night. Flavonoids are particularly important for diabetics, whose eyes and kidneys are prone to damage as a result of poor capillary circulation. An additional benefit from PCOs is their ability to help reduce the risk of heart disease.

Supplements

If you want to take a supplement of citrus flavonoids, one that contains a standardized mixture of 1–3g of flavonoids is likely to be more effective than mixed citrus flavonoids in which the levels of individual flavonoids, such as rutin and hesperidin, can vary.

Drug interactions

Naringin, one of the citrus flavonoids, interacts with a number of drugs, including estrogen and caffeine, to prolong or heighten their action. If you take prescribed medication, check with your doctor before taking supplements that contain naringin or grapefruit juice. PCO supplements are also available and have no known side effects.

Fill your diet with powerful plants

Carotenoids

Green, red, and yellow vegetables and fruits, such as carrots, pink grapefruit, watermelon, apricots, mangoes, yams, tomatoes, red and green cabbage, kale, spinach, berries, and plums

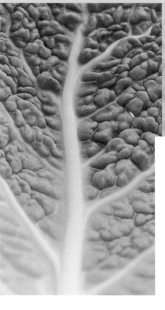

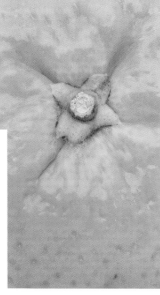

Flavonoids

Citrus fruits, berries, onions, parsley, legumes, green tea, and red wine

Legumes, grains, and seeds

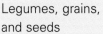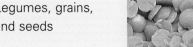

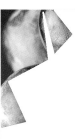

PCOs: Cherries, raspberries, strawberries, red grapes and blueberries

EATING FOR A **HEALTHY HEART**

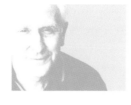

Heart disease is the number one killer in many developed countries. Major causes are the development of atherosclerosis (fatty deposits in the major arteries) and elevated blood pressure. The good news is that atherosclerosis is often directly caused by an unhealthy diet and other lifestyle choices (see smoking, page 70; exercise, page 50; and stress control, page 84), and it can be reversed. Adopting a healthy lifestyle can also reduce high blood pressure, but not in all cases. Some people can only accomplish this through medication.

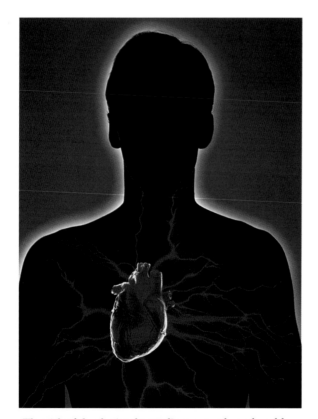

The risk of developing heart disease can be reduced by eating a healthy diet and exercising regularly.

The healthy-heart diet is based on the Optimum Diet (see page 15). Particularly important areas are:

■ Reducing consumption of saturated fats and cholesterol.

■ Eating plenty of high-fiber food.

■ Maintaining weight at the correct level for your height (see page 43).

■ Cutting down or eliminating caffeine intake and drinking plenty of water.

Fat: getting the balance right for a healthy heart

Primates of roughly the same size as human beings, such as the gorilla and orangutan, eat diets that contain about 1.5 percent of food from animal sources. It has been suggested that this amount would be the ideal for humans. This is a rather extreme view, but there is no doubt that the amount of food from animal sources in developed

A Scottish secret

Porridge for breakfast is good for the health of your heart. The 3g of soluble oat fiber found in every bowl of porridge helps to keep cholesterol levels low. If your cholesterol level is already high, you can reduce it by up to 23 percent by eating porridge regularly, with low-fat milk. For each percentage point drop there is a 2 percent decrease in the risk of developing heart disease. Porridge contains less fiber than oat bran, but it lowers cholesterol more effectively, probably because it is rich in unsaturated fats.

countries is often too great (more than 50 percent for many people). One reason is the quantity and nature of the fat contained in domesticated animals. Beef, for example, contains 25–30 percent fat compared with 4 percent in wild animals. Beef fat is mostly saturated, and contains virtually no omega-3 fat (see page 20), which makes up about 4 percent of the fat in wild animals. Good sources of unsaturated fats are given on page 19.

Your heart needs carbohydrates

Whole grains, legumes, and fresh fruit and vegetables are extremely important for a healthy heart. They are rich in vitamins and minerals, including the antioxidant vitamins C and E, and the minerals calcium, magnesium, and potassium, all of which help to keep blood pressure under control. Fruit and vegetables are also the richest sources of flavonoids and carotenoids (see page 32), and some, such as onion, garlic, and celery,

may be particularly good for the heart. Unprocessed carbohydrate foods are rich in dietary fiber (see page 22), which helps to lower cholesterol levels and is also helpful for weight control.

The daily diet should include several servings of wholegrain or higher fiber foods, starting with breakfast because people who begin the day this way have, on average, the lowest cholesterol levels. In addition, 3–5 servings of vegetables and 2–4 servings of fruit should be eaten each day, raw or lightly cooked. These are rich in potassium and naturally low in calories and salt, which increases blood pressure in some people.

Protein and your heart

Protein intake should be restricted as suggested in the Optimum Diet, and most of it should come from vegetable sources. So-called white meats, however, such as skinned turkey, and white fish contain low levels of fat.

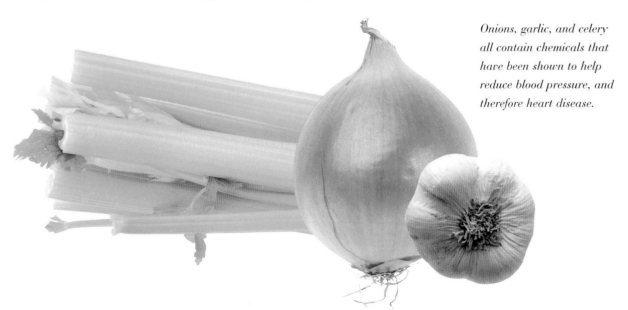

Onions, garlic, and celery all contain chemicals that have been shown to help reduce blood pressure, and therefore heart disease.

EATING FOR A **HEALTHY GUT**

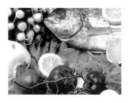

Indigestion is a term often used to describe the feeling of a mild stomach upset, or a burning sensation behind the breastbone. Once your doctor has assured you that you do not have a serious condition, it is worth trying some self-help. A common cause of indigestion is overeating, so small regular meals can help. Relief can also be obtained by reducing the intake of fried food, chocolate, coffee, alcohol, or sodas, and by smoking less. If you have been told that you have a hiatal hernia or acid reflux disease and your indigestion is worse at night, you should avoid eating late in the evening. Your condition may also be helped by raising the head of your bed by about 4 inches (10 cm).

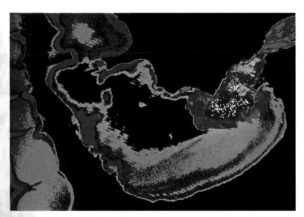

Heartburn can be attributed to disturbances in the production of stomach acid and other digestive secretions.

Food combining

Many people believe that their digestion and general health have been improved by separating starchy foods from protein. Unfortunately, there is no known physiological reason for this improvement, but you can adopt the following rules if you want to see if food combining works for you.

Basic rules of food combining

Fruits	Proteins	Vegetables	Starch
Fruit should be eaten on its own. This can be a single fruit snack or fruit-only meal, in which case fruit of the melon family should not be eaten with other fruit.	Only eat one protein at each meal and choose nonstarchy vegetables, such as greens, salad leaves, or zucchini, for example, to go with it.	In the food-combining diet there is great emphasis on eating a large quantity of vegetables.	Dishes made from starchy vegetables, such as potatoes, can be eaten with any other vegetables. Although starchy foods often contain protein, they seem to be more easily digested if no other protein is present.

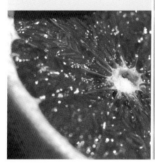
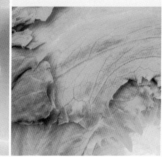
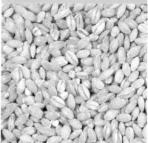

Irritable bowel syndrome (IBS)

This common problem should be diagnosed by a doctor to exclude other rarer conditions that may have similar symptoms. Once you know IBS is your problem you can improve your symptoms by:

Eating more fiber: adding wheat bran is the easiest way to increase fiber, but it is not always the best choice (see food intolerance, right), and too much bran may reduce the absorption of minerals. Follow the Optimum Diet (see page 15) and gradually increase the fiber in your diet by eating more unprocessed whole food, including grains, fruit, vegetables, and legumes in particular. (Always drink more water as you increase your fiber levels.) This allows time for the digestive system to adapt, but this approach should be stopped if you experience diarrhea.

Eating less sugar: even if you do not have the yeast syndrome (see page 72), symptoms can be caused by the muscles in the wall of the intestine becoming less active or stopping altogether when refined sugar is eaten.

Better stress management (see page 84).

Looking for possible food intolerance: this is not a true allergy, so normal allergy tests are not helpful. However, if you write down everything you eat over two or three days, the food or foods to which you are intolerant are usually the ones you eat most often. It is worth totally excluding these foods for a few days to see if your symptoms improve. Even if you do not notice much improvement, your symptoms may get much worse when you start to eat normally again, indicating that you are intolerant to them (see also page 77).

The foods that commonly cause food intolerance are grains (especially wheat), and those containing milk (including whey). Food intolerances change over time, and you will usually find you can reintroduce the problem food(s) after a few months, provided you do not then eat them too often.

HEALTHY SKIN AND HAIR

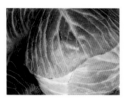

Skin and hair need constant nourishment and they are often the first to suffer if your diet is inadequate. To avoid this, adopt the Optimum Diet (see page 15), with plenty of water-rich fruit and vegetables to prevent constipation and maintain a clear, fresh complexion. Even if you choose to add supplements to your diet; these should be taken in addition to, not instead of, a good diet (also see pages 24–27 for cautions).

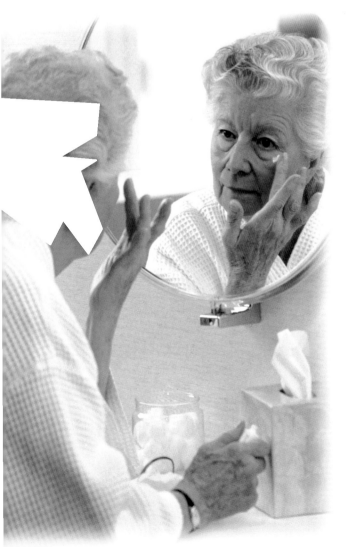

Vitamins A, C, E, and selenium

These antioxidant nutrients help to counteract the premature aging of the skin that is often caused by exposure to the sun, tanning beds, cigarette smoke, and other pollutants. In addition, the diet should contain plenty of carotenoids and flavonoids, especially PCOs (see page 32) because these also help to keep the skin healthy. And don't forget sunblock with a minimum SPF of 15, and wear a wide-brimmed hat between 10 a.m. and 3 p.m. when in the sun.

The B vitamins

The cells of skin and hair divide constantly so they need a good supply of B vitamins. Doctors and nutritionists very often look for changes in the skin to detect deficiencies of B vitamins; inadequate intakes of vitamins B_1, B_2, B_3, and B_6 can all be detected in the skin. Biotin is another B vitamin that is of particular importance to healthy skin. It may also help to keep the nails strong and prevent premature graying of the hair.

A healthy diet, such as the Optimum Diet, can help to keep the skin looking clear and provides moisturization from within.

There is no recommended daily intake for biotin because it is present in many foods, and the bacteria in the intestine also make it. However, deficiency can occur if you take antibiotics for a long time, eat a very low-calorie diet, or eat raw eggs regularly, as all these factors can limit the absorption of biotin. Biotin deficiency is an uncommon cause of hair loss in women.

Silicon

The mineral silicon is thought to be important for supple skin and strong connective tissue, bones, fingernails, and hair. It may also help to prevent graying of the hair. The main food sources of silicon are vegetables, whole grains, and seafood, and it is a major ingredient of food supplements manufactured from alfalfa and the herb horsetail (*Equisetum*).

Sulfur

Sulfur, dubbed the "beauty mineral," is another nutrient essential for healthy skin, hair, and nails. It is found in many foods, but especially in proteins, legumes, onions, garlic, and vegetables of the brassica family, such as cabbage, broccoli, and kale, as well as Brussels sprouts, turnips, or kohlrabi. Although it is not known how much we need to obtain each day, sulfur is extremely unlikely to be deficient in a diet that contains adequate protein.

Copper

Copper (see page 30) is needed to make melanin, the pigment that gives color to skin and hair, and it is also present in the connective tissues. Dietary deficiency is thought to be relatively common when too many refined foods are eaten, but the use of copper plumbing in soft water areas greatly increases your copper intake.

Supplementation can be tricky because high levels can result in zinc deficiency (and vice versa), and are toxic. However, a multimineral preparation is likely to be safe, if supplementation is needed.

Essential fats

Dry skin is more common at 50+. Even the liberal application of moisturizers will not help the problem if the diet contains insufficient essential fats (see page 20). Although only relatively small amounts are needed, they can be lacking if the diet has a very low fat content.

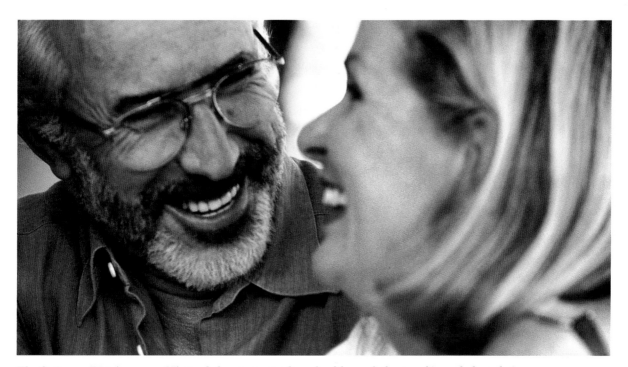

The Optimum Diet (see page 15) can help ensure you have healthy and glowing skin and glossy hair.

THE SENSES

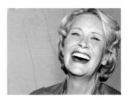

The ability to see and hear is precious, and the ability to taste adds greatly to the pleasure of eating. The fact that what we eat at 50+ may influence the health of these senses at 80 is being recognized by some nutritionists. This is another reason to adopt the Optimum Diet (see page 15), as it contains nutrients that may protect all of our senses.

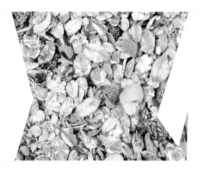

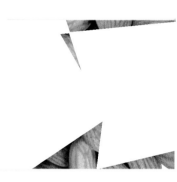

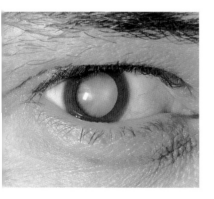

Eating the Optimum Diet may delay, or even avoid, the formation of a cataract within the lens of the eye.

Age-related macular degeneration (ARMD) and cataracts

ARMD and cataracts are common causes of failing sight, and both can be the result of damage caused by free radicals, and the relative deficiency of other essential nutrients.

Some protection may be provided by:

- Eating plenty of fruit and vegetables, especially legumes, which are rich in sulfur, dark green leaves (spinach in particular), red and yellow vegetables for carotenoids (see page 32), berries for flavonoids (see page 32), whole grains and nuts for vitamin E, and citrus fruits, kiwi fruits, and other rich sources of vitamin C.

- Eating a range of zinc-rich foods. Animal foods, such as lean meat, fish, and eggs, are good sources of zinc and are easily absorbed. Plant sources of zinc include the germ and bran of grains, as well as nuts and seeds. However, plant sources of zinc tend to be less well absorbed.

■ Avoiding fried, grilled, and rancid foods, which are sources of free radicals.

■ Avoiding cigarette smoke: smokers who have quit smoking have an increased risk of developing ARMD for up to 15 years after stopping.

■ Taking supplements of PCOs (see page 33).

Glaucoma

Glaucoma is a condition in which the pressure in the aqueous humor (the fluid that fills the chamber of the eyes) is higher than normal, causing damage to the optic nerve. Glaucoma requires medical diagnosis and treatment. Although it can result in blindness, dietary changes may be of some preventative value. This is especially true for those whose relatives have developed glaucoma, which can be an inherited condition.

Nutrients that may provide some protection are vitamin C (citrus fruits, kiwi fruits, parsley, and other green vegetables), flavonoids, especially PCOs (see page 32), magnesium (in dark green vegetables), and chromium (in whole grains, meats, shellfish, and vegetables).

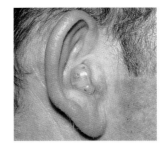

Avoiding deafness may not be possible, but modern hearing aids are inconspicuous and powerful.

Hearing

Loss of hearing has a number of causes, few of which will respond to a nutritional approach. Because it is often part of the aging process, however, food containing vitamin C (citrus fruits, kiwi fruits, parsley, and other green vegetables) and the B vitamins (see page 24) may be helpful as they maintain tissue health. Supplements containing the B vitamins help some people whose deafness is caused by Ménière's disease.

Taste

Loss of taste can be the result of zinc deficiency, which will also cause the appearance of white spots on the nails. Zinc deficiency can occur in people with a small appetite or who eat a vegetarian diet (see ARMD and cataracts, left). There is also some evidence that the absorption of zinc becomes less efficient with age. Some conventional medications can also cause loss of taste.

Blueberries

Blueberries have been used for food and as folk medicine for centuries. They are a rich source of PCOs (see page 32) and can be eaten as berries or prepared as a food supplement. However, excessive intake over a long period of time may compromise the immune function.

Possible benefits

■ Improvement of night vision and quicker recovery after exposure to glare

■ Prevention and treatment of glaucoma

■ Protection against the development of ARMD and cataracts

■ Prevention of diabetic retinopathy

■ Reduced symptoms of arthritis and gout

■ Improved sugar control in diabetes (under professional guidance)

ADULT-ONSET
DIABETES

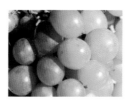

Adult-onset, or type 2, diabetes starts rather insidiously in middle age or old age, and may not be diagnosed until the eyes or kidneys are irreversibly damaged. In fact, it is often discovered by an ophthalmologist during a routine eye test. To some extent adult-onset diabetes is an inherited condition and if your parents, grandparents, or other members of your family have developed the condition it is a good idea to ask your doctor about testing you for it.

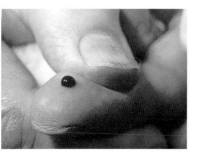

The finger-prick test enables people with diabetes to monitor their blood sugar levels accurately at home.

Who develops adult-onset diabetes?

You are more at risk of developing adult-onset diabetes if you are overweight. In many people, obesity causes the cells of the body to become resistant to the action of insulin (a hormone that removes sugar from the blood and transports it into the body's cells). This means sugar levels in the blood stay high because the insulin is unable to remove it. Juvenile diabetes, or type I, which starts at a younger age, is different because it is caused by a lack of insulin.

Where the extra fat is stored in overweight people can also provide a clue to the risk of developing adult-onset diabetes. Doctors have observed that those people most at risk carry their weight around their middle. This so-called "apple shape" is more likely to precede diabetes than the "pear shape," in which extra fat is stored around the buttocks and thighs.

What you eat may also increase the risk of adult-onset diabetes. Resistance to insulin by the cells is aggravated by a lack of chromium, which can be deficient in a diet that contains too many refined foods, such as white flour, bread, and sugar. In addition, too much fat in the diet may reduce the absorption of chromium from food. Chromium deficiency is a particular problem in the United States, where there are low levels of the mineral in the soil.

Lowering the risks of diabetes

The recommended diet for people with adult-onset diabetes, or those who are at risk of developing it, is based on the Optimum Diet (see page 15) including, where necessary, eating for the right weight (see right). Adequate vitamin and minerals are essential because they can help to reduce the complications of diabetes.

There is much research to support the view that adult-onset diabetes is related to a low fiber intake, so a high-fiber diet is recommended for both treatment and prevention. The best way to increase the fiber in your diet is to eat wholegrain cereals, whole fruits and vegetables, including their skins where appropriate, nuts and seeds, and, perhaps most important of all, legumes. Legumes are rich in fiber and chromium, and they are digested very slowly, thus avoiding rapid changes in the level of sugar in the blood. Fiber supplements appear to be less effective in reducing the risks of diabetes than eating the fiber in food.

In addition to a good diet, increasing the amount of exercise you get can be highly beneficial and may even reverse the onset of diabetes, especially when any excess pounds are also shed. Chromium is one of the minerals that is lost in perspiration (see page 60), and it is important to ensure an adequate daily intake.

Good sources of chromium

■ Most fruits and vegetables

■ Brewer's yeast

■ Beef

■ Cheese

■ Egg yolks

■ Grapes, grape juice, wine

■ Wholegrain cereals and their unrefined flours

■ Hard water (in some areas)

Eating for the right weight

Even if you have never had a problem maintaining your optimum weight, you may find this becomes less easy at 50+. The main problem is the gentle decline in what scientists call the metabolic rate, which is simply a measurement of the rate at which the body burns up energy. The decline can be offset by getting exercise (see Chapter Two).

The Optimum Diet (see page 15) can be adapted for weight control:

■ At least 70 percent of your food should come from fruit, vegetables, wholegrain cereals, and beans. Eating a large green salad (with a fat-free dressing) or fat-free vegetable soup 10–15 minutes before a meal can blunt hunger.

■ Be strict about your fat intake. Fat is high in calories and does not send messages of fullness and satisfaction to the brain. Read food labels critically: "85 percent fat free" means that every 100g (3½oz) of the food contains 15g (½oz) of fat.

■ Avoid refined sugars and alcoholic beverages. Eat whole fruit rather than drinking fruit juices, or choose vegetable juice.

■ Drink plenty of water: the feeling of hunger is sometimes simply thirst.

■ If you need to make major changes to your diet, do this gradually to allow your digestive system to adapt.

In addition to good diet, increasing the amount of daily exercise you do can be highly beneficial in preventing and treating diabetes.

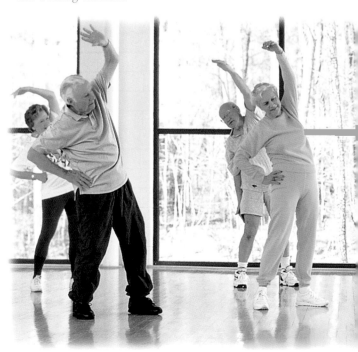

EATING FOR
PAIN-FREE
JOINTS

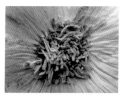

Painful and stiff joints were once considered "normal" for many people at 50+. Today, practitioners of natural medicine believe that up to 70 percent of people with one of the various forms of arthritis can reduce, or even eliminate, pain by making dietary changes. For many people, relief comes from removing certain foods from their diet and also increasing foods that are known to ease joint inflammation. Unfortunately, there is no one diet that will help everyone, but some changes that have been found to be helpful are shown below.

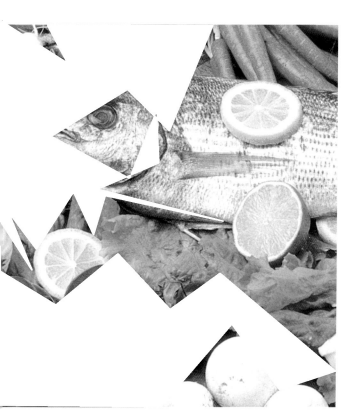

You can reduce the chemical additives that you eat by basing your diet on fresh organically grown fruit and vegetables.

Changing your diet

Many people are helped if they follow the Optimum Diet (see page 15) and also eliminate chemical additives. The Optimum Diet provides vital nutrients for the body to use as it tries to heal damage in the joints, the immune system, and the digestive system. Food intolerance (see pages 37 and 77) is often associated with painful joints, and it is best to avoid eating large amounts of any one food-type. Try to reduce the amount of salt you eat and ensure that you eat plenty of fiber, from a number of sources, as suggested on page 22, rather than just wheat bran.

Eliminate chemical additives as rigorously as possible by cutting out the following foods:

■ Caffeine: tea, coffee, and chocolate/cocoa, including decaffeinated products. If you normally drink large amounts, cut down gradually over a couple of weeks to avoid withdrawal symptoms. Decaffeinated tea and coffee are rarely completely caffeine free, and can contain chemical residues.

- Sugar and all artificial sweeteners: many condiments contain sugar, so it is important to read food labels.

- All sodas, and any other manufactured carbonated drinks.

- Manufactured foods that contain chemical additives, such as colorings, preservatives, flavor enhancers, flavorings, thickenings, emulsifiers, stabilizers, etc. These include margarine, bacon, ham, corned beef, sausages, and smoked foods.

- Foods that make the intestine more "leaky" (see page 72), including very heavily spiced foods and raw pineapple and papaya. If possible, gradually reduce aspirin and nonsteroidal anti-inflammatory drugs because they also damage the gut.

- Produce that has been chemically sprayed should be avoided if possible. However, it is more important that whole grains and fresh fruit and vegetables make up 65–70 percent of your diet, so if you eat nonorganic produce wash it thoroughly.

Follow the above recommendations for at least a month. You may then feel that your symptoms have improved sufficiently for you to adopt this way of eating in the long term. However, if your symptoms have not changed at all, you may be intolerant to some of the foods that you are continuing to eat, or you may need to talk to a nutritionist. (See page 77 for food intolerance).

Some helpful foods

Different medical traditions have found that certain plants may relieve the pain of inflamed joints. These include spices such as ginger, cayenne pepper, paprika, and the pigment curcumin, found in turmeric. Herbalists recommend garlic, the root and leaf of dandelions, nettles, celery seed, alfalfa, mint, and bitter greens such as mustard, watercress, and the many varieties of endive or chicory that are becoming easier to

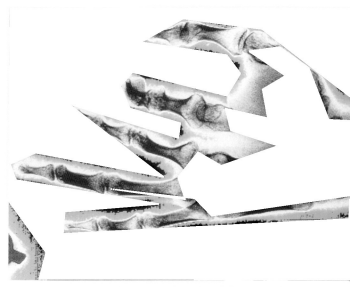

The oils in fish can help to ease the pain of rheumatoid arthritis by reducing inflammation in the joints.

obtain, either as leaves or seeds for cultivation. The red and blue colors of berries and cherries signify the presence of flavonoids with many healing properties, including pain relief.

Oily fish and flaxseed (linseed) oil contain the beneficial omega-3 fatty acids, which can help inflamed joints, but are in short supply in the diet of most people in developed countries. Limited amounts of omega-3 oils are also present in cod and halibut liver oils, which contain vitamins A and D as well (see cautions on pages 24 and 26).

Oily fish

Eating two or more portions each week of the following can help your heart as well as your joints:

- Anchovies

- Herring

- Mackerel

- Rainbow trout

- Salmon

- Sardines

- Tuna.

I'D LOVE A **HEALTHY DIET,** BUT...

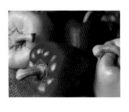

It is very easy to simply buy a bottle of vitamin and mineral supplements and continue to eat the same old diet in the hope that illness or chronic fatigue will happen to someone else. They will certainly happen to someone, and can, unfortunately, happen to those who have tried really hard to live a healthy life. However, if everyone adopted a healthy diet some doctors, at least, would be short of work.

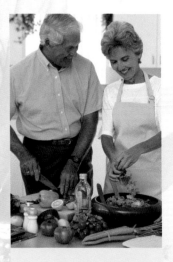

"You are what you eat..."

If you can't cook, haven't the time, or never want to cook again

A healthy diet can be a cordon bleu extravaganza, but most of us want to have enough to eat, at the time we want to eat it, with a minimum of effort. Initially, this may take a little planning, but once healthy eating is habitual you will find that it takes no extra effort.

Breakfast

Do not skip breakfast. It is perhaps the most important meal and should contain a wholegrain cereal, high in fiber, which helps to keep cholesterol levels low. Try these suggestions:

- A piece of fruit and/or ³/₄ cup (6 ounces) of fruit or vegetable juice, plus one of the following:

- A bowl of low-sugar wholegrain cereal

- Porridge with skim milk: oatmeal soaked overnight cooks quickly and can be sweetened with dried fruit,

OR have a breakfast blender (see below), which takes a couple of minutes to make and drink, but can be prepared the night before and stored in the refrigerator overnight if you really do not have time in the morning.

Lunch

A large salad, including a vegetable protein, such as beans or brown rice left over from the previous evening, or a few sunflower or pumpkin seeds, plus wholewheat bread or a crispbread, spread with hummus or sugar-free peanut butter,

OR vegetable soup that contains lentils or brown rice, plus wholegrain bread spread with low-fat cottage cheese,

OR a packed lunch based on wholegrain bread with a protein spread, such as hummus, low-fat cottage cheese or peanut butter, and salad vegetables (washed the previous evening), such as tomato, cucumber, celery, raw carrots, bell peppers, etc. Or just take the vegetables and buy a wholegrain, low-fat sandwich

PLUS a piece of fruit, and/or low-fat yogurt and/or a few nuts.

Dinner

Start with a salad, or vegetable sticks with a bean dip or guacamole, or soup, or a platter of steamed fresh vegetables. Then have a protein dish, such as lean meat or fish with lightly steamed vegetables,

OR pasta/rice/quinoa with a sauce based on tomatoes or other vegetables, and containing some other vegetable protein such as beans, tofu or corn, or animal protein such as chicken or shrimp.

OR a turkey or shrimp stir-fry, with vegetables and served on noodles.

FINISH with fresh fruit or low-fat yogurt.

Snacks

Fresh or dried fruit, a few nuts or seeds, vegetable sticks prepared from carrots, celery, cucumber, bell peppers, etc.

The breakfast blender

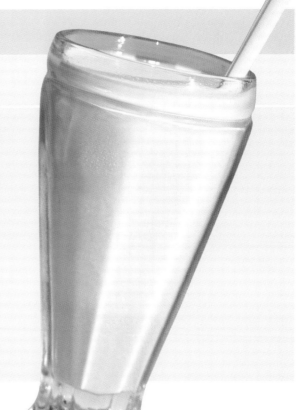

Combine the following in a blender:

3 or 4 different fruits, including, if possible, fresh or frozen berries and/or stoned cherries

1 to 2 tablespoons of flaxseeds: start with a small amount because this is a natural laxative, or 1 tablespoon of cold-pressed flaxseed oil

½ cup (110ml) fat-free yogurt

2 tablespoons of oat bran, rolled oats, or oatmeal

FRESH FRUIT AND VEGETABLES

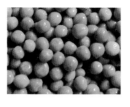

Fresh fruit and vegetables are an important part of every diet since they are rich in vitamins, minerals, phytonutrients (see page 32), and fiber (see page 22). Most of them contain plenty of water and virtually no fat, so they are economical in calories, too. North American guidelines advise eating 3–5 portions of vegetables every day and 2–4 servings of fruit. Few Americans achieve this, but it is not difficult if you replace all your snacks with fruit and have salad and vegetables at midday and in the evening.

Fruit

Fruit is generally popular as a snack or as a convenient second course to finish a meal. Most fruits are sweet, juicy, nutritious, and easy to digest. For convenience, have washed fruit ready to hand. Take some along with you if you will need a snack where the only other food available to buy is likely to be candy, chocolate, or cakes, or where washing fruit would be impossible.

Most fruit should be eaten fresh and uncooked. Fresh frozen fruit is the next best nutritionally, and dried fruit is often more nutritious than canned fruit. Fruit that is gently stewed in its own juice can be easier to digest, and is helpful when chewing is a problem.

Vegetables

Vegetables are an important source of carbohydrate in the diet. Most vegetables are best eaten fresh and raw, but many people are unable to digest sufficient quantities of raw vegetables. Some, such as potatoes, have to be cooked anyway and others release more nutrients when cooked. Cooked carrots, for example, are a richer source of beta-carotene than raw carrots.

The best cooking methods for vegetables are baking or lightly steaming, as some vitamins and minerals leach into the water when vegetables are boiled. These nutrients can, however, be conserved if you use the cooking water to make soup, gravy, or other sauces. Both dried and canned vegetables lose vitamins during processing, but freshly frozen vegetables retain most of their nutrients.

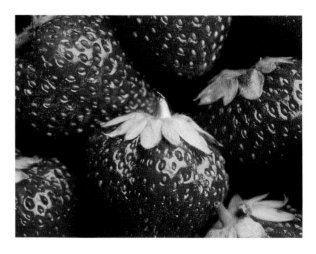

Choosing fruit and vegetables

When possible, choose organically grown produce: it requires a minimum of washing, and does not need to be peeled. Nonorganic produce has usually been treated with chemical pesticides and waxes, and is best washed thoroughly and peeled.

Unfortunately, the vitamins in fruit and vegetables can be lost in storage and, along with certain minerals, in cooking. Maximize the nutrients in your fruit and vegetables by:

■ Shopping for produce more than once a week, choosing a shop with a good turnover.

■ Eating produce ripe in its natural season: it is generally nutritionally superior to produce that has been picked early and artificially ripened. In temperate climates some storage of food is essential for the winter months.

■ Washing salad and other leafy greens after buying them, allowing them to dry and storing in a plastic container or bag in the vegetable compartment of the refrigerator.

■ Keeping fresh herbs in a little water in the refrigerator.

■ Storing mushrooms in a paper bag in the vegetable compartment of the refrigerator.

■ Storing fruits, potatoes, tomatoes, onions, and garlic in a cool, shady place, rather than the refrigerator. Potatoes should be stored in the dark.

Juices

Freshly juiced fruit and vegetables are particularly rich sources of vitamins and minerals, but they are low in the natural fiber that is so essential for health. Fruit juices, in particular, contain large amounts of sugar, and should always be diluted with the same volume of water. Some vegetables, such as carrot, and beets, also contain sugar, and their juices are best diluted with other vegetable juice, such as celery, spinach, or cabbage.

If you eat no animal protein

Choose from at least two of the following food groups each day:

Whole grains: wheat, rice, rye, corn etc.

Legumes: beans, peas, lentils etc.

Seeds: sunflower, sesame, pumpkin etc.

Nuts: almond, hazel, walnut, Brazil, macadamia etc.

Vegetarian diets

Vegetarian diets may be chosen for ethical reasons, or simply because they are thought to be healthier. However, vegetarians who eat dairy products and rely too much on cheese sometimes eat more animal fat, which is predominantly saturated fat, than meat-eaters (see page 19). There are even some vegetarians who do not eat vegetables! The Optimum Diet (see page 15) applies to vegetarians as much as to anyone else.

The list of protein portions (see page 18) clearly shows that there is plentiful protein in whole grains, nuts, legumes, and seeds. Even potatoes contain an adequate proportion of protein by weight. However, although all animal sources of protein are complete for human needs, the protein in plants is usually incomplete, apart from soybeans. Vegetarians, therefore, should eat some animal or soy protein each day, such as cheese, milk or yogurt, or at least two types of plant protein (see box above).

Vegetarians who never eat animal protein (vegans) can be deficient in zinc, iron, and copper if they choose a diet that contains too many refined foods, or if they have small appetites. If necessary, a supplement should be taken.

Iodine deficiency has been reported among vegans, but this can easily be remedied by eating kelp, or another seaweed. Vitamin B_{12} does not occur in plant foods, and vegans should obtain it by eating fortified cereals or brewer's yeast.

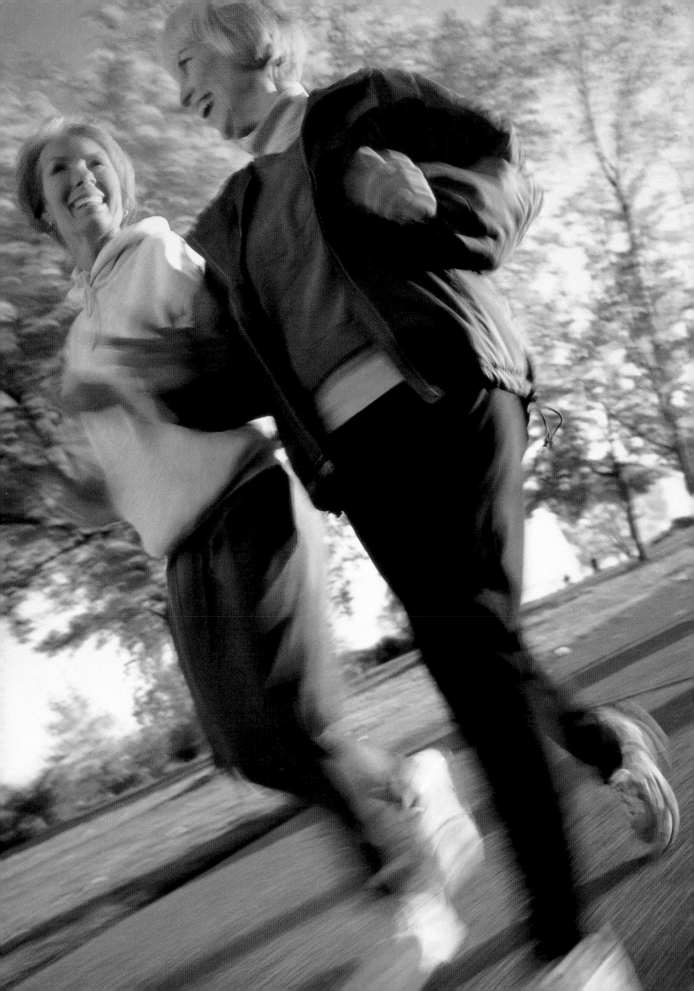

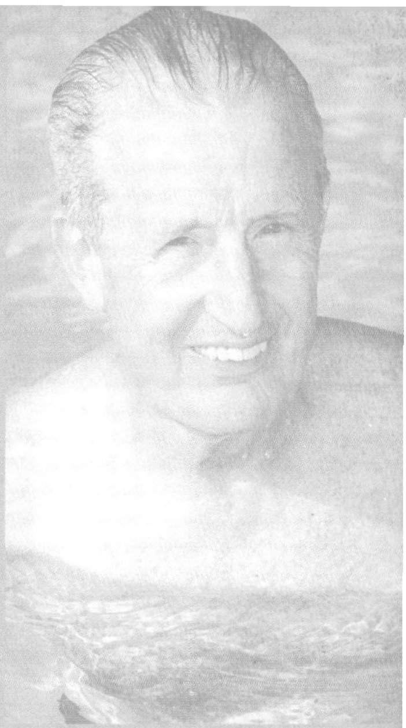

Chapter Two

EXERCISE:
WHERE, WHY, AND HOW

Many of the current 50+ generation are not as fit as they should be. During the second half of the twentieth century almost everyone came to benefit from the use of a car and labor-saving domestic appliances in the home. Many people drive instead of walking to do their errands, or spend too much time watching television or surfing the web. The resulting lack of exercise and physical exertion has been one of many factors contributing to the epidemic of the diseases that doctors label "degenerative," such as heart attacks, obesity, adult-onset diabetes, and osteoporosis.

"The wise, for cure, on exercise depend."

John Dryden (1631–1700)

HOW
REGULAR
EXERCISE

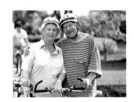

HELPS

Most people make financial plans for their retirement, but they often neglect to invest in their continuing physical well-being. They assume wrongly that nothing can be done about the gradual loss of physical fitness that starts at about the age of 30. The truth is that people who don't stay in shape age more quickly than those who look after themselves, and an inactive lifestyle hastens the aging process.

Positive action

There are major benefits to keeping in shape. For most people, at least some investment in regular exercise will be required if they are to keep their mind, heart, muscles, and bones in good shape. Even if exercise does not prolong your life, it is likely to improve its quality, and 50+ is not too soon to take the need for regular exercise seriously.

It should be possible to undertake a beneficial amount of exercise without major changes to your routine. If you exercise regularly you should continue with what you enjoy. However, before commencing a new exercise regime at 50+, it is a good idea to check that your doctor has no objections. This is essential if you have any health problems.

Getting started

Congratulations! You have decided to begin exercising regularly, and you are now raring to go. However, if you have been sedentary you should ease yourself into your exercise program slowly, partly to avoid problems with your muscles and joints and partly to allow your heart time to adapt to working a little harder. Start by setting aside 10 minutes three or four days a week. If you have had a heart attack or other illness, your doctor may suggest that you start with 3–5 minutes three

times a week. Gradually extend your exercise time as you become stronger.

As a rough rule of thumb, to build up to a full program you will need about a month for each year of sedentary living, or longer if you have had any health problems.

How much is enough?

Your breathing provides a guide as to whether your exercise is challenging you enough, or too much. You should be breathing more rapidly than usual, but not be so out of breath that you cannot talk. A more accurate measure of exercise's effect on your heart is to take your pulse, either at the wrist, or just in front of the upper part of the ear at the back of the cheekbone. Count your pulse beats for 10 seconds and multiply by 6 to give the rate per minute. Your heart will benefit from any regular exercise, but the greatest benefit occurs when it is beating at between 70–85 percent of the maximum rate for your age (see table, right) for 15–20 minutes, or for longer when you are fit.

If your heart rate is higher than the target for your age, you are overdoing it and should slow down. As you get into shape you will find that you keep your heart rate safely within the target range.

Listen to your body

Do not take these figures absolutely literally: try to respond to what your body is telling you. Exercise should not cause discomfort, and if you experience pain in the chest, jaw, or neck, you should consult your doctor. Be prepared to slow down in cold or windy weather, or when going up a hill. Remaining excessively tired an hour or more after finishing exercise may indicate that you are attempting too much. Exercise should be enjoyable: it is not a punishment.

Warming up and cooling down

Starting your exercise slowly will give time for the temperature in your muscles to rise, so they become more elastic and less vulnerable to injury. Stretch your muscles five minutes into the warm-up.

Let your body return to its normal temperature gradually by slowing the pace of your exercise a few minutes before stopping. This will help prevent the stiffness that can occur if you stop suddenly.

What to wear

Start with loose, comfortable clothing that absorbs sweat and washes easily. The only real essential is a pair of high-quality shoes designed specifically for the type of exercise you are doing. Women also need a comfortable bra that provides support.

What about the weather?

In hot and humid weather drink plenty of water before, during, and after exercise. If possible, exercise early in the morning or during the evening. Dress warmly in cold weather and wear a hat. If you have had any heart problems ask your doctor whether it is safe for you to exercise in cold or windy weather.

Increasing your exercise

Once you comfortably manage the starting level you have chosen for your exercise, increase your exercise time by 2–5 minutes per session. Rest days are important so only exercise five days a week.

Table of maximum and target heart rates per minute for your age

Age	Maximum	Target for greatest benefit for the heart (70–85% of maximum)	Target for a fat-burning program (see page 55) (60% of maximum)
50	170	119–145	102
55	165	116–140	99
60	160	112–136	96
65	155	109–132	93
70	150	105–128	90
75	145	101–123	87
80	140	98–119	84
85	135	94–115	81
90	130	91–110	78
95	125	87–106	75
100	120	84–102	72

EXERCISE YOUR **HEART**, **LUNGS**, AND **CIRCULATION**

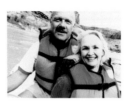

Not so long ago people were told to rest after a heart attack. Today, there is ample evidence that a gradual exercise program can extend and improve the quality of your life after a heart attack, and may even help prevent another one from occurring.

The heart is a muscle, and like every muscle in the body it needs oxygen from the blood. Exercise increases the number and size of the blood vessels in all the muscles of the body and it reduces the likelihood of a clot forming in one of the heart's blood vessels, which is one cause of a heart attack. Blood vessels also become more elastic as you exercise, so they are less likely to rupture under pressure. Exercise increases the efficiency of the heart muscle, so that it pumps blood more efficiently through the body.

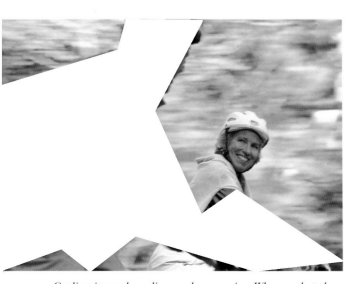

Cycling is good cardiovascular exercise. When undertaken three or four times a week, it can help with weight loss.

The lungs

Exercise enables your lungs to function more effectively. A gentle, gradually increasing exercise program can help to overcome the problems, such as the fear of not being able to breathe deeply enough, caused by asthma and emphysema. Mild emphysema is a common lung condition in which the alveoli (air sacs) of the lungs become overextended and less efficient, usually as a result of smoking or pollution. Although exercise does not reverse the underlying damage to the lungs, it can increase the amount of activity that can be undertaken. Even people with severe emphysema, who become breathless after the slightest effort, can benefit and, as a result, maintain or regain some independence.

EXERCISE AND **OBESITY**

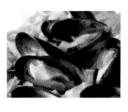

In general, obese people get less exercise than people of normal weight, but it is uncertain whether this is a cause of obesity or its result. Either way, regular exercise is a must if you want to lose weight, and is more effective when combined with a lower-calorie diet. Moderate to intense exercise can also reduce your appetite.

You should restrict weight loss to 1–2 lbs (0.75–1 kg) per week; a greater loss than this after the first week or two suggests that you are losing muscle. Once you have achieved your target weight you should continue to exercise to avoid regaining the weight you have lost.

As a calorie-restricted diet progresses, the body naturally tends to conserve energy and weight loss therefore slows or stops. This is counteracted by exercise, which increases the rate at which energy is used both during exercise and for several hours afterward.

The best exercise for weight loss is of long duration (45–60 minutes per session), and of low intensity (about 60 percent of your maximum heart rate, see page 53). Good examples are walking or cycling, at least three or four days a week. Swimming seems to be less effective.

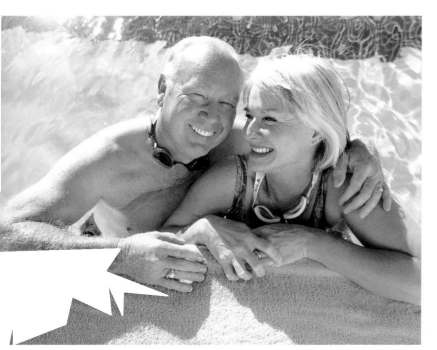

Exercise and adult-onset diabetes

Adult-onset diabetes is most likely to affect people who are overweight, but it can often be entirely reversed when the program described above results in weight loss. If you have any of the eye complications of diabetes, you should avoid exercise that jars your body (unless your doctor recommends otherwise). In this case, swimming is a good choice.

Swimming is an ideal form of exercise for diabetes, as it does not jar the body.

EXERCISE AND
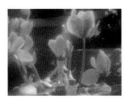

OSTEOPOROSIS

Osteoporosis, which literally means "porous bones," results from the loss of calcium and the other minerals that are essential for strong, dense bones. Although osteoporosis is generally thought to be a condition that mainly affects women, it is now being diagnosed with greater frequency in men.

Doing an hour of moderate exercise three times a week can be sufficient to prevent osteoporosis. Exercise has also been shown to increase bone density even when osteoporosis has already commenced. However, if you have developed osteoporosis you should seek professional advice and exercise gently at first to avoid fracturing any bones. Exercise should be continued for life because any benefits to your bones are lost within a year of stopping.

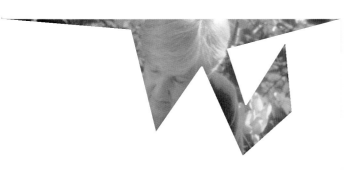

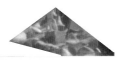

Gardening is a good, inexpensive form of exercise and can be as gentle or as strenuous as you like.

Exercising outdoors brings an added benefit. Exposing the skin to the sun for short periods without sun-blocking creams enables the body to make the vitamin D that is needed to help calcium be absorbed by the body. It is best to avoid the midday sun, which is more likely to burn the skin and cause skin cancer.

What sort of exercise is best?
Exercise for osteoporosis should stretch, compress, bend, and twist the bones. This means that many everyday activities, such as gardening, housework, and even carrying the groceries home, are all valuable for the arms and upper body. Walking, dancing, jogging if you are fit enough, and going up and down stairs all benefit the bones of the spine and the legs, including the

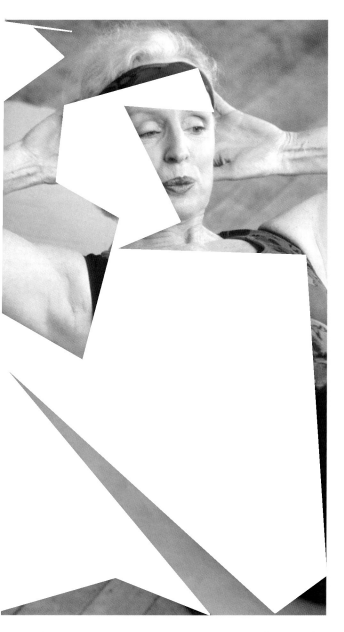

Stretching your muscles and moving your joints on a regular basis can help to reduce stiffness.

because it limits intake of protein and refined sugar, both of which can deplete calcium. In addition, a generous intake of green leafy vegetables provides plenty of calcium, boron, magnesium, potassium, and vitamin K, all of which help to strengthen the bones.

Other bone preservers

Giving up smoking, restricting alcohol intake to one drink a day for women and two drinks a day for men, (see page 71) and avoiding carbonated drinks, which are high in phosphate, all help to preserve your bones. You should avoid antacid medicines that contain aluminum and the use of aluminum skillets, because the aluminum dissolves in acidic food and can interfere with calcium absorption.

Supplements to consider

- Calcium: (Caution: avoid calcium supplements from dolomite, bonemeal, or oyster shell, unless the manufacturer guarantees they are free of lead contamination.)

- Vitamin D: especially during the winter or if you are housebound. Avoid high doses, which may adversely affect magnesium levels.

- Magnesium

- Vitamins B_6, B_{12}, and folic acid: for the elderly who often have a dietary deficit.

- Silicon: may be helpful in the treatment of established osteoporosis.

- Phytoestrogens: these estrogenlike substances from plants have been used in many conditions that are now treated in orthodox medicine by estrogen. Found in soy products such as tofu, and soy milk, their benefit for osteoporosis is not yet scientifically established, but they are thought to be helpful.

hips, which are among the commonest bones to be fractured. For elderly people any type of daily activity, including chair exercises (see page 63), can be beneficial because calcium leaves bones very rapidly when a person is immobile, even for a few days. Cycling, swimming, and yoga are of limited benefit for counteracting osteoporosis.

Can dietary changes help?

At 50+ the differences in bone density between meat-eaters and vegetarians becomes more marked, probably because calcium is lost from the bones more slowly in vegetarians. The Optimum Diet (see page 15) will help to prevent osteoporosis

EXERCISE AND THE **JOINTS**

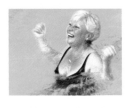

Stiffness in the mornings and the occasional painful joint become more common at 50+ and one of the causes may be lack of exercise. Even if you develop one of the many forms of arthritis, regular exercise should be continued whenever possible. It helps by contributing toward a healthy heart and maintaining normal weight, mental alertness, better sleep, and optimum balance and posture. More specifically, exercise keeps the joints fully mobile and relieves muscle tension – which can add to joint pain – while maintaining strength in the muscles surrounding the joints.

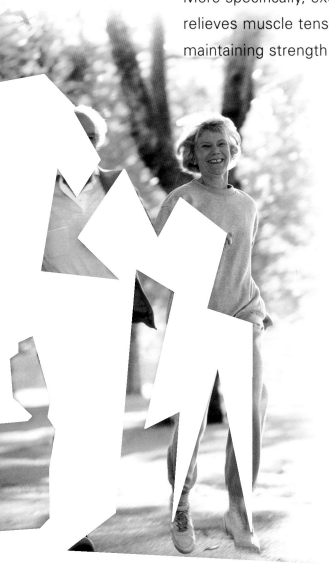

Choosing your exercise

Choose activities that do not strain or jar your joints. Select your footwear carefully: good-quality supportive shoes are particularly beneficial because they absorb some of the jolt that may be transmitted to the joints when the heel hits the ground. Swimming and water aerobics are good choices for people with painful joints because the buoyancy of the water removes much of the body weight from the joints.

How much exercise is safe?

You should not continue with any exercise that causes you pain or discomfort, but it is worth trying it again a couple of weeks later when your muscles are stronger. If any discomfort you experience after exercise lasts longer than two hours you have probably done too much, and should cut back. If you have arthritis you should not exercise an acutely inflamed and painful joint. Moving it gently within the range of movement that is relatively pain-free, however, can reduce stiffness.

Exercising with a friend or partner can be an encouragement on the days when you are tempted to stay at home.

EXERCISE AND THE **MIND**

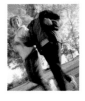

Few people can avoid some degree of stress in their lives. The body is designed to react to stress and sudden physical danger by producing a burst of epinephrine, which prepares us for "fight or flight." Neither reaction may be appropriate or possible as we get older, so the epinephrine surges through the body, elevating blood pressure and causing physical tension.

Exercise

A safe way to use up the excess epinephrine is a good workout. There is ample scientific evidence to support the psychological benefits of exercise, but the reasons are more complex than just using up spare epinephrine.

Regular exercise is like a mini-vacation and much of the benefit may simply be a result of having time to think or to take your mind off your problems. On a physical level, exercise improves the circulation, which delivers oxygen to all tissues, including the brain. When senile patients in a veterans' hospital in the United States were given pure oxygen, their scores in a standard memory test improved by as much as 25 percent.

Depression and anxiety

For many people regular exercise can help reduce the negative feelings of depression and anxiety. This may be because in exercising you are physically active, and the sense of achievement can help you to feel better about yourself and more in control of your life. Repetitive movement, as in walking, jogging, or cycling, can be very relaxing because it temporarily suspends the need to make decisions. The companionship and friendship of competitive sports can help overcome feelings of isolation.

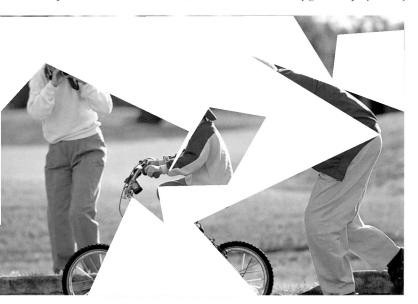

Spend time with your grandchildren as they will keep you physically active and mentally alert.

EXERCISE: **ENERGY** AND DIET

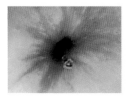

Once you start doing more exercise, it is important to continue with the Optimum Diet (see page 15). You can refuel your body's stores of readily available carbohydrate (glycogen) after your exercise period by eating a meal that is rich in unrefined carbohydrate. If you feel shaky and a bit wobbly during exercise, it is likely that your sugar level has dropped too low. Eating a snack that contains unrefined starchy food two hours before exercise can help to prevent this: avoid caffeine and sugar, even fruit sugar, especially if this is taken as juice. If the problem persists, carry a banana or apple in your pocket for use during energy drains.

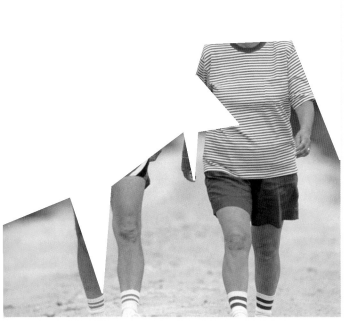

Walking is a very beneficial form of exercise; it is good for reducing stress and doesn't cost anything.

When people of normal weight start an exercise program, they may find they can maintain a higher calorie intake without gaining weight, and therefore maintain an adequate intake of minerals and vitamins more easily. Overweight people do not usually increase the amount of food that they eat when they start exercising. Hopefully, the extra energy they are using will come from their fat stores, and they should continue to eat a diet that is rich in unrefined carbohydrates and low in fat.

Water and sweat

As you exercise, your muscles warm up and you will start to sweat; this is the body's way of controlling its temperature. Loss of fluid through perspiration is best replaced by drinking water, before, during, and after exercise. Caffeine and alcohol should be avoided because they increase fluid loss by increasing the amount of urine produced. Minerals, including sodium, potassium, magnesium, and chromium, are lost in perspiration, but the Optimum Diet is rich in all of them.

EXERCISE: ALMOST EVERYONE CAN **WALK**

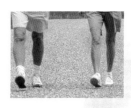

Walking is often the most convenient way to begin getting more exercise. Almost everyone can walk and you can start with a very gentle program. If there is no convenient circular route from your home, just walk for half your allotted time before turning around and going back home again. Walking costs nothing and can be introduced gradually into anyone's daily activity. Best of all, perhaps, walking can reduce stress, because just the rhythm of putting one foot in front of the other is relaxing.

It is important to walk briskly enough to increase your heart rate (see page 52). However, if you have been very sedentary or are overweight you may find that your heart rate is increased even when you are walking slowly. Do not be discouraged; just give yourself time.

Seven ways to walk more

■ Get off your bus one stop earlier or park a little way from the office and walk the rest of the way to work.

■ Use the stairs rather than the elevator or escalator. Start off by walking down, and when your legs are stronger, start walking up as well.

■ Don't use the car for short trips, such as going to the corner store or mailing a letter.

■ Fit a walk into your lunch hour.

■ If you don't own a dog, offer to exercise a friend's dog.

■ Encourage a routine of family walks during the weekend.

■ Choose a time of day that rewards you. Some people like the early morning; others find they sleep better after an evening walk.

Safety

If you are walking at night, walk facing the traffic and wear light-colored clothing, preferably with reflective stripes.

TAKE **FIVE** MINUTES

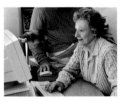

If you sit at a desk for long periods or are confined to a chair at home, try the following gentle exercises to stretch your muscles. If you have severe arthritis or osteoporosis ask your doctor if the exercises are safe for you before you begin. Initially do the exercises once a day, but as you become stronger, repeat each exercise more often and hold the positions for longer.

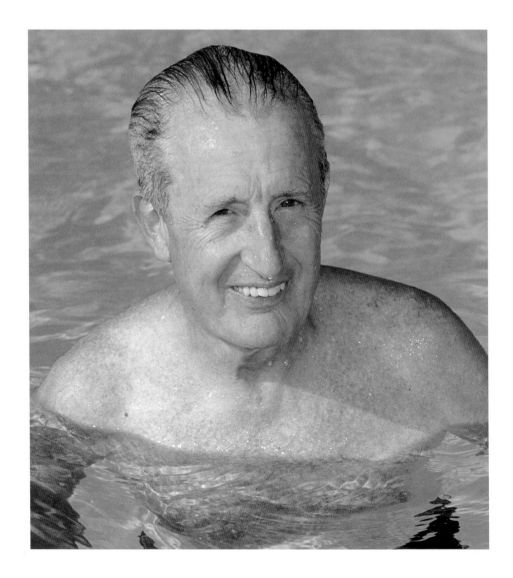

The exercises

Arms

1. Keeping your back straight, shrug your shoulders and then roll them around to the back, then down, then forward, and rest. Repeat the exercise moving in the reverse direction.

2. Hold your right arm straight out to the side with your palm downward. Bend your right elbow and bring your hand around until it is just below your chin. Reach out to the side again. Repeat once. Do the same exercise with the left arm.

3. Stretch your right arm forward, level with your shoulder, palm upward, and then bend the elbow and lightly touch your right shoulder. Straighten your arm and repeat once. Do the same exercise with your left arm.

4. Tuck your elbows into your sides with the palms facing each other, and then bend your wrists so that the tips of the fingers almost touch. Repeat twice. Then move your hands around in circles one way, then the other.

Legs

1. Sit upright as far back on the chair as possible. Straighten your right leg. If necessary, support yourself by holding the sides of the chair. Hold it for 2–3 seconds, then put your foot back on the floor. Do the same on the left, and then repeat once.

2. Sit with both your feet flat on the floor, then lift the heel of your right foot. Hold it for 2–3 seconds, and then place the heel back on the floor. Do the exercise with the left foot. Repeat once. Then lift the front of the right foot, leaving the heel on the floor and stretching your toes. Hold this for 2–3 seconds before putting your toes back on the floor. Do the same with the other foot. Repeat once.

3. Still sitting, cross your legs, right over left, and move the right foot to make a circle first clockwise, then counterclockwise. Repeat with the left foot.
(Do not attempt this exercise if you have had a hip replacement operation.)

Trunk

If you have had a hip replacement or have osteoporosis of the spine ask your doctor or physiotherapist if these exercises are suitable before you try them.

1. Place your hands on your hips, turn from your waist to look toward the right, hold for 2–3 seconds, relax, and turn to the left. Repeat.

2. Face forward with your hands in your lap. Keeping your back straight, rotate your trunk clockwise twice. Pause, then repeat the exercise in a counterclockwise direction.

Neck

Start and finish each exercise looking straight ahead.

1. Lower your chin as far as it will go comfortably, then lift it gently back again. Do not bend your head backward. Allow your head to nod gently up and down two or three times.

2. Turn your head to the right as far as it will comfortably go and then to the left, and return to the starting position. Repeat twice.

3. Drop your head sideways gently toward your right shoulder, and then toward your left shoulder. Keep your shoulders relaxed. Repeat twice.

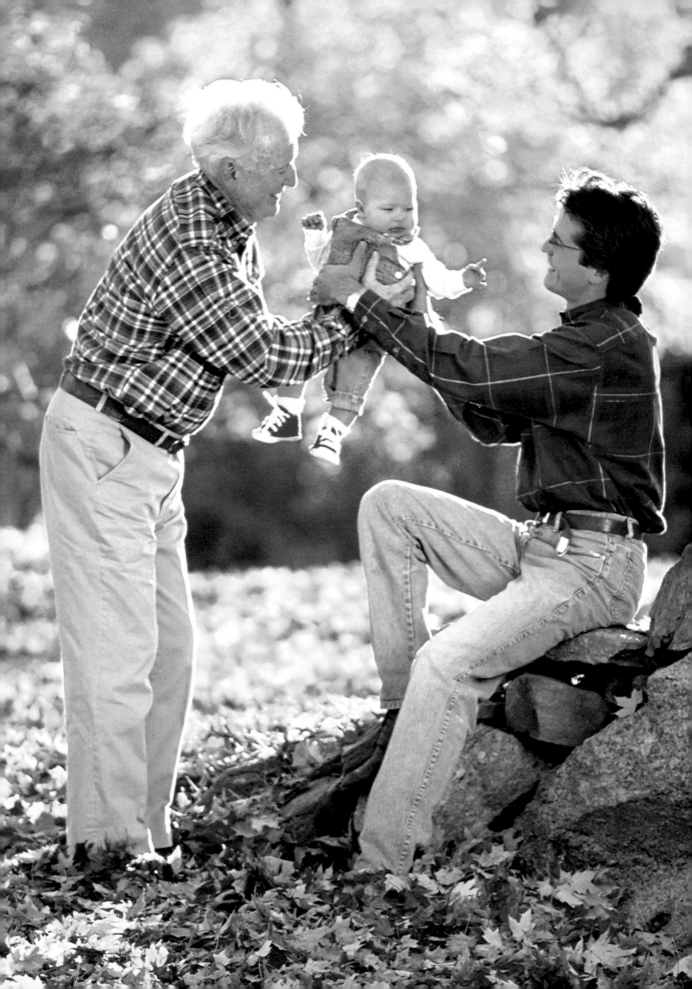

Chapter Three

A HEALTHY
IMMUNE
SYSTEM

A healthy immune system protects the body against infections, allergies, and the development of cancer. There is growing evidence that the immune system can play a major role in preventing, or at least minimizing, a number of other ailments, such as arthritis and some heart conditions. At 50+, therefore, nurturing the immune system should be a priority if you wish to remain healthy.

"Our immune system is the most dynamic body component in determining our state of health or disease."

Elson M. Haas, M.D.

THE IMMUNE SYSTEM

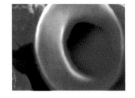

A major task of the immune system is to protect the body from infections caused by bacteria, viruses, fungi, and other microbes. The first lines of defense are the skin and the mucous membranes lining the nose, mouth, digestive system, and other parts of the body. Additional protection is provided by chemicals contained in the mucus and other secretions, such as saliva and tears.

Additional defenses are mobilized once a microbe has entered the body. These defenses include the white blood cells, antibodies, and chemicals that act as messengers to alert and control the immune system. These immune system components have the ability to distinguish between the cells of the body that they defend and the cells of invading microbes, which contain foreign proteins that have to be destroyed. The immune system is also able to "remember" certain infections, such as those from the viruses causing measles or mumps. The antibody response when the same virus is met again is therefore very quick, so a second illness is normally prevented.

The proteins in food are also foreign proteins, but the digestive system breaks them down into their building blocks, the amino acids. In a healthy person these are absorbed either individually or in small groups, so that the immune system is not usually triggered into action. In

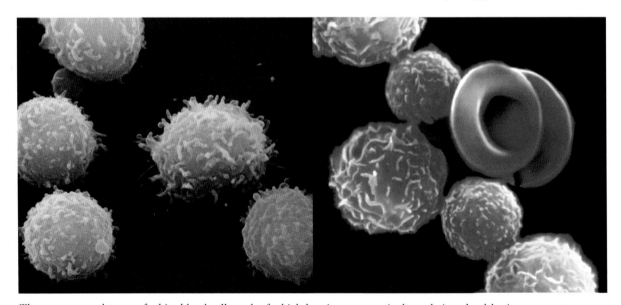

There are several types of white blood cell, each of which has its own particular role in a healthy immune system.

addition, when digested food is absorbed into the bloodstream it is transported to the liver, where any harmful substances that have survived the digestive process are detoxified, before the nutrients are released into the rest of the circulation.

As part of the body's internal repair and maintenance capacity, the immune system also provides protection by removing aging or damaged cells from the body before they can do harm. These include potentially cancerous cells that may have been damaged by free radicals, or cells that have resulted from imperfect cell division.

Clinical ecology

In the 1940s, Dr. Theron Randolph, a young doctor with an allergy practice in Chicago, began to draw the attention of doctors to illnesses that he believed had been triggered by environmental factors. His particular concern was the increase in the amount of chemicals from industry, agriculture, and other activities that were being found in the air and in food and water. He was one of the founders of a medical movement that is often called clinical ecology (see also page 143).

Today, it is generally accepted that gross chemical contamination is harmful, but the effects of exposure to chemicals at low levels remains controversial. Clinical ecologists use the term chemical sensitivity to describe the adverse reaction that some individuals appear to experience when exposed, even at a very low level, to toxic chemicals. Although some of these reactions are true allergies, many of them result from the failure of the body to detoxify harmful chemicals. In practical terms, however, the symptoms are often similar, as are the measures that will provide protection.

Loving your liver

The liver plays a major role in both the immune system and the process of detoxification. Almost two quarts of blood pass through the liver every minute, and it filters out bacteria, viruses, dead cells, cancer cells, and other foreign and dangerous particles. It also breaks down chemicals, including drugs and pesticides, that have entered the body and which may cause damage. In a healthy person, the liver performs these functions efficiently, but it can become overwhelmed, especially if it has been damaged, for example, by alcohol.

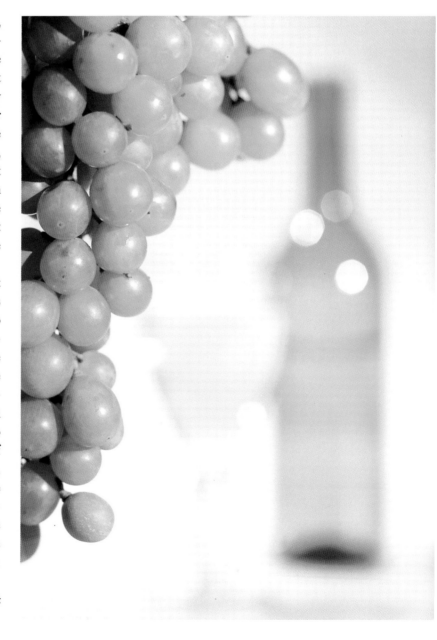

Alcohol abuse can cause your liver to work inefficiently, or even to cease functioning.

Strengthening the immune system

At 50+ the immune system is likely to have sustained some damage from illness, exposure to pollution, and from deficiencies in the diet. There is also increasing evidence that both physical and mental stress can suppress the effectiveness of the immune system. However, the body has a great capacity to heal itself, and you can support this process by reducing stress (see Chapter Four), by getting regular exercise (see Chapter Two), and by ensuring you get adequate rest: try to sleep for at least seven hours a night.

Nourishing the body, and therefore the immune system, can be achieved if you follow the guide-lines for the Optimum Diet (see page 15), paying particular attention to the following:

■ Eat ample vegetables, especially greens.

■ Keep added chemicals to a minimum, including salt (see also Eating for Pain-Free Joints, page 44), and avoid unnecessary medication. Choose organic produce when possible.

■ Eat regularly, and make sure that you are obtaining enough protein (see page 18), since it is needed for the repair and replacement of the components of the immune system.

■ Avoid being overweight by exercising regularly; this can suppress the immune system.

■ If you choose to drink alcohol, do so in moderation (see page 71), and stop smoking (see page 70).

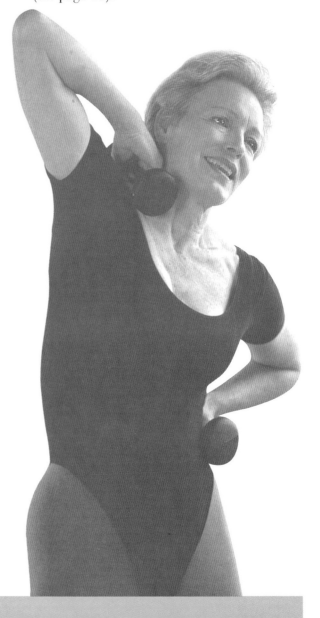

Coenzyme Q$_{10}$

This enzyme, which occurs naturally in the human body, supports the immune system by enhancing the body's ability to protect itself from many conditions, including heart disease, and from some of the effects of prescribed medications. Unfortunately, the amount produced tends to decline with advancing age just at the time that it is most needed. A good diet helps the body to manufacture coenzyme Q$_{10}$, but you can consider a supplement. The usual dose is up to 30mg/day, but higher doses are often recommended and you should seek professional advice if you are uncertain.

Ensuring a low-toxin environment

You may believe that your home is a safe place in which to live, and that in your work environment the law protects you from exposure to harmful chemicals. Yet, neither may be true. The US Environmental Protection Agency has reported that "indoor air pollution in residences, (and) offices...is...one of the most serious potential environmental risks to health." In the UK, the Building Research Establishment recommends that houses should have a complete air change every two hours. Conditions reportedly resulting from contact with indoor pollution include asthma, chronic sinus infections, headaches, insomnia, anxiety, fatigue, and joint pain. In the 50+ age group, many of these conditions are attributed to getting older, and yet they may be totally avoidable.

- Reduce your use of pesticides both inside the house and in the garden.

- Avoid wearing outdoor shoes in the house because they will track in pesticides and other chemicals.

- Avoid added chemicals in food (see page 45); eat organic produce when possible and consider fitting a water filter on your faucet.

- Hang new and recently dry-cleaned clothes in the fresh air for a few hours, so that any chemicals remaining in the fabrics have a chance to disperse.

- Choose solid wood furniture, or seal composite bonded materials with a low-toxicity sealant.

After gardening, remove your shoes before entering the house.

Tips for detoxifying your home

- Air your home every day by opening your windows for 15 to 20 minutes once or twice a day, and decrease the use of chemicals: indoor pollutants include paints, cleaning agents, solvents, dyes, glues, and household sprays.

- Avoid buying carpets treated with fungicides and permanent stain-resistant chemicals.

- Have your gas appliances and boiler or furnace serviced regularly, and if you have an open fire keep the chimney swept. Avoid portable oil and gas heaters.

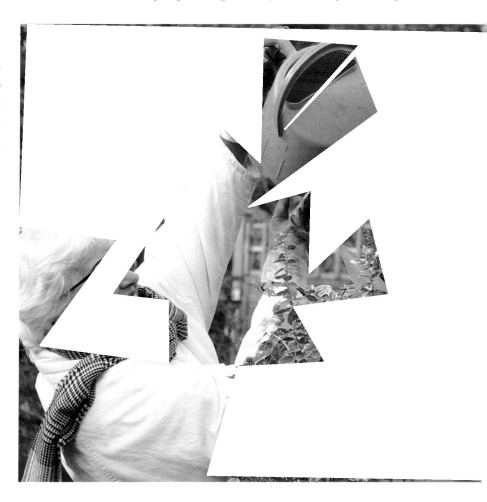

BREAKING **HABITS** AND **ADDICTIONS**

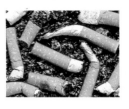

Tobacco smoke contains not only at least 50 substances that can cause cancer, but also thousands of other chemicals that are known to damage the heart and circulation. Therefore, the biggest boost you can give your immune system is to stop smoking and avoid the company of those who still do.

Smoking is an addictive habit and, as with all addictions, stopping is not easy, but it can be done. Millions of people have stopped, and the scientific evidence suggests that "just stopping" is the most successful method. If you have been a heavy smoker, however, it is probably wise to cut down gradually over a few days or weeks, or to use patches or chewing gum that contains nicotine for a few weeks.

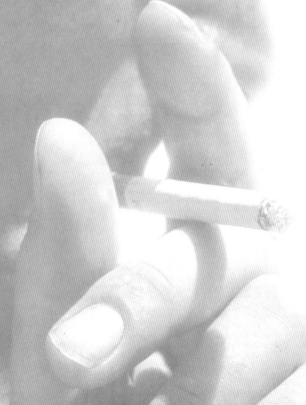

The following tips might help you to quit smoking:

- Write down your reasons for not smoking, and read the list every day.

- Set the day and tell your friends! Don't make it more difficult than necessary by choosing a day when temptation will be high, such as the day of a party.

- The night before you intend to stop, throw away any unsmoked cigarettes, empty the ashtrays, and air out the house well.

- Plan substitutes: have raw vegetable sticks already prepared in the refrigerator to occupy your hands and mouth when you have an urge to smoke.

- Try deep breathing exercises, or go for a walk when you have the urge to light up.

- Take one day at a time: the urge to smoke will eventually leave you.

- Join a support group.

- For a few weeks at least, avoid situations that you associate with smoking.

- Put aside the money you save by not buying cigarettes and spend it on something pleasurable, but try to avoid high-calorie rewards.

Alcohol

Alcohol is a toxic substance that can suppress the immune system in a number of ways – not least by diverting the liver, which detoxifies alcohol as a priority – from some of its other tasks. The presence of alcohol in the body can reduce the effectiveness of some of the specialist cells of the immune system, causing drinkers to be more prone to infections than nondrinkers. Direct contact with alcohol can damage the cells that line the mouth, gullet, and stomach, increasing the risk of developing cancers in these areas. In the intestine, the presence of alcohol can interfere with the absorption of nutrients, which are important for the function of the immune system.

You will obtain 0.5oz of alcohol from:

1oz of 100 or 110 proof liquour

1½ oz of 80 proof liquor

8oz of dark beer

12oz of regular beer

Reduce your alcohol intake by drinking nonalcoholic drinks or diluting your drinks with a mixer.

Aids to safe drinking

- Limit your intake of alcohol to one drink a day for women or two drinks for men, and aim to have two alcohol-free days a week.

- Quench your thirst with a nonalcoholic drink.

- Dilute your drink with a mixer.

- Lower the level of alcohol in your blood: delay its absorption by eating low-salt carbohydrates, such as bread or raw vegetable sticks.

- If you have drunk too much alcohol, take some vitamin C and a B-complex vitamin supplement and drink plenty of water before going to bed.

- Never replace a meal with alcohol.

- If you feel that you cannot do without alcohol, you may have an alcohol problem and should consider seeking professional advice.

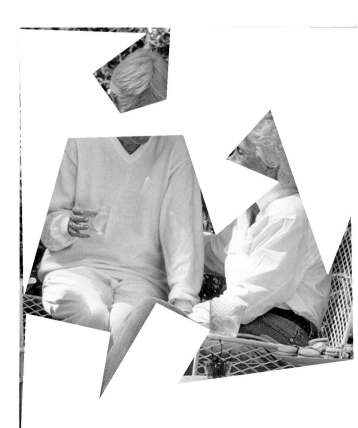

INFECTIONS **OLD** AND **NEW**

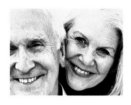

Mankind has always suffered from infections. In the past couple of centuries, however, there have been many triumphs over infectious diseases. These include the eradication of smallpox and – in developed countries, at least – improvements in hygiene, as well as the introduction of various vaccines and more effective drugs. We are also gaining a better understanding of how to nourish and bolster our immune systems. As a result more people are surviving into old age.

But it would be a mistake to become complacent. Researchers have known for several decades that microbes can mutate, and we are often now faced with bacteria that are resistant to current antibiotics. Old problems thought to have been largely overcome, such as tuberculosis, are returning, and new problems, such as acquired immune deficiency syndrome (AIDS), have emerged. The full name for AIDS is a chilling reminder that a virus can somehow learn to undermine the immune system.

The yeast syndrome and immune suppression

In the 1980s some doctors began to recognize that a pattern of symptoms was occurring among patients who had received either frequent or prolonged treatment with antibiotics. The symptoms include various degrees of fatigue, headaches, memory problems, allergies, and other disorders of the immune system, depression, and an aversion to cigarette smoke and other chemicals, such as perfumes and household cleaning agents. Digestive disturbances that also often occur include irritable bowel syndrome (see page 37), bloating, and intolerance of certain foods (see page 77).

It has been assumed that the symptoms of this condition, which has been labeled the "yeast syndrome," are caused by an excessive amount of *Candida albicans* (see box, right) in the digestive system. Unfortunately, there is as yet no scientific proof to support this assumption, and some doctors prefer to use the term "fungal-type gut dysbiosis," which means an intestinal dysfunction caused by a yeast.

The yeast syndrome might cause a "leaky gut," (see page 45) which allows the absorption of inadequately digested proteins. Because these are foreign proteins they stimulate the immune system into action, and divert it from tackling chronic infections, such as recurrent sore throats, herpes infections (cold sores), and fungal infections of the skin, such as athlete's foot and ringworm.

Because the diagnosis of yeast syndrome remains controversial within the medical profession, getting advice is not always easy. If you think that you suffer from the yeast syndrome it is important to consult someone who is properly qualified, such as a doctor, naturopath, or nutritional therapist, before embarking on treatment. The strict dietary restrictions that may be involved can themselves cause ill health.

Reducing the chances of developing yeast syndrome

- Avoid antibiotic and steroid medicines, unless they are absolutely necessary.

- Adopt the Optimum Diet (see page 15) and be sure to include plenty of garlic and yogurt.

- Avoid refined sugar and limit the amount of fruit juice that you drink.

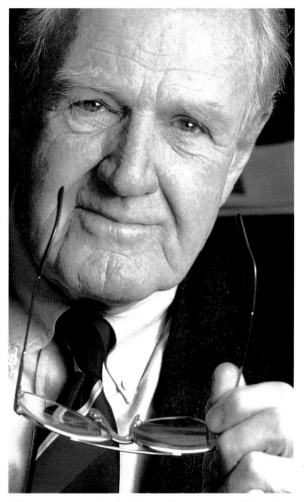

We can now combat infectious diseases more effectively, so more people are surviving into old age.

Candida albicans

This yeast, which lives in the intestine (and the vagina in women), is normally quite harmless. However, like many microbes it can cause infection if it becomes too widespread, as has long been known to happen when the immune system has been damaged by diseases, such as cancer, or by certain drugs, such as steroids. Many doctors have found difficulty in accepting that *Candida* can be responsible for the yeast syndrome, which usually occurs in people without serious illness and who have not been taking drugs known to suppress the immune system. All the same, treatment can transform the quality of life for some people.

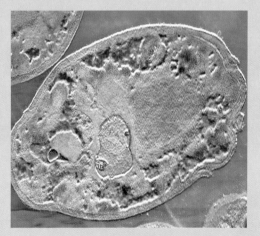

Enlargement of a cell of Candida albicans.

CANCER
AWARENESS

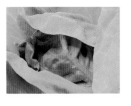

Although cancer can have specific and known causes, such as cigarette smoke or exposure to high doses of radiation, the majority of cancers are likely to result from a series of complex factors, many of which are poorly understood. A tendency toward cancer can be inherited, but a strong family history of the disease is merely one factor among many, including being 50+, that should spur the active avoidance of carcinogens and a nurturing of the immune system.

Give your immune system a rest by minimizing exposure to cigarette smoke, which is associated with nearly all lung cancers, as well as some cancers in the upper digestive system, pancreas, and bladder. Also try to reduce your exposure to other potentially harmful chemicals (see pages 69 and 143).

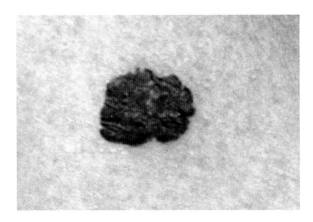

Malignant melanoma is a particularly dangerous type of skin cancer.

Overexposure to the sun causes most types of skin cancer. The skin can be protected by applying sunblock, but this interferes with the production of vitamin D in the skin. Fortunately, vitamin D is stored in the body, and sufficient amounts of the vitamin can be obtained by exposing the skin daily, without sunblock, to the sun during spring and summer for about 15-20 minutes. In the south of the US you should avoid the midday sun. In the north of the US, the sun in winter is not always strong enough to make vitamin D in the skin and it is wise to ensure that you obtain some from your diet or to take a supplement.

The cancer awareness diet

The particular features of the Optimum Diet (see page 15) that may help reduce your risk of developing specific cancers are:

- Eating 3–5 servings of vegetables and 2–4 servings of fruit every day may reduce the risk of cancer of the digestive system and, in women, of breast cancer. It is thought that vegetables of the cabbage family are particularly beneficial, such as broccoli, Brussels sprouts, kale, bok choy, mustard greens, kohlrabi, and turnips. Other valuable vegetables are lettuce (especially the dark green varieties), spinach, and parsnips. (See also Plant Power, page 32.)

- Limiting the amount of red and processed meats that you eat to about 3oz (90g) per day on average. This level is thought to reduce the risk of cancers of the rectum and colon, without your losing out on iron and the other essential minerals that are present in meat.

- Limit or avoid smoked, salt-cured, pickled, fried, and barbecued foods. These methods of treating food introduce chemicals, which, if eaten in excess, may increase cancer risks.

- Avoiding obesity (see page 43). This is associated with an increased risk of breast and uterine cancer, and possibly also some intestinal cancers.

- Increasing the fiber in your diet. This may reduce the risk of cancer of the rectum, colon, breast, and, possibly, the pancreas. Try to obtain fiber from eating a variety of fruits, vegetables, legumes, and wholegrain cereals rather than by adding fiber supplements, which may reduce the absorption of minerals. Nuts and seeds are rich in fiber, but high in calories, although the fat they contain is mostly unsaturated (see page 19).

- Limiting alcoholic drinks to the recommended levels (see page 71).

Overexposure to the sun causes most skin cancers.

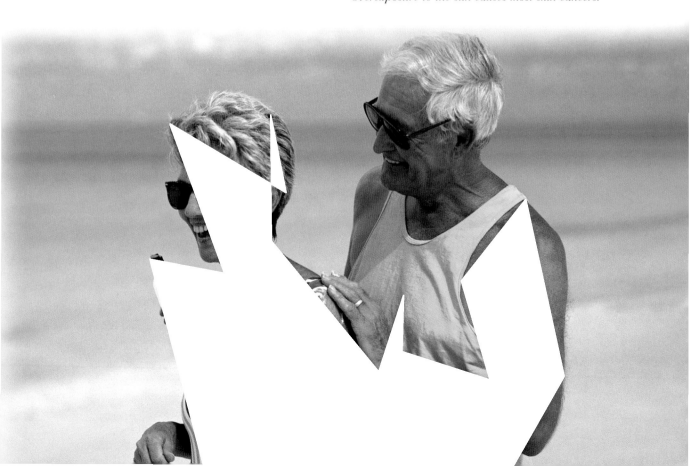

ALLERGY: THE IMMUNE SYSTEM IN OVERDRIVE

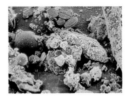

Allergies are best regarded as abnormally excessive reactions to otherwise harmless substances. However, allergies are becoming much more common for reasons that are not well understood. The orthodox approach to allergies is to suppress the symptoms with antihistamine or steroid-based medication, but these can cause side effects, so many people turn to natural therapies for help. Homeopathy (see page 168) and herbal treatment (see page 161) are very often effective treatments for hayfever, house dust allergy, and skin reactions to food, such as hives (urticaria).

Prevention is another approach. One way is to avoid the substances, known as allergens, to which you overreact. This can be difficult when the allergens that affect you are numerous or have not been identified with certainty.

Preventing allergies

Some doctors believe that you can benefit from even a modest reduction in exposure to the allergens that affect you, especially when this reduction is coupled with other lifestyle improvements, such as:

■ Eating the Optimum Diet (see page 15), to keep your immune system healthy and working effectively.

■ Avoiding the chemicals that are added to food (see pages 45 and 75) and minimizing your exposure to other chemicals (see page 69). In this way the burden on the immune system is

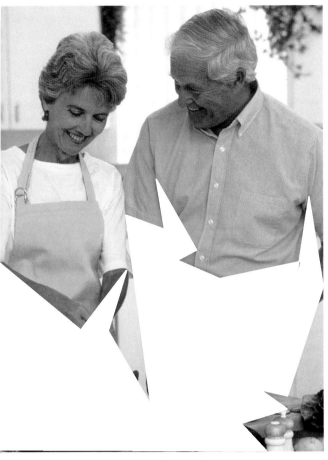

A healthy diet should include 3–5 portions of vegetables and 2–4 portions of fruit each day.

reduced, so it is better able to react normally to other substances and avoid allergic reactions.

■ Paying attention to psychological health (see Chapter Six), as there is a growing awareness among scientists that our emotional and immune systems are closely connected.

Food allergy

True food allergies are normally lifelong reactions to a particular food or foods. The foods are usually easily identified and can, in theory, be avoided. Allergic reactions to food include digestive upsets, a runny nose and watery eyes, and the itchy rashes that are sometimes known as "hives," or urticaria.

More seriously, food is one cause of a condition that doctors call anaphylaxis. This is a potentially life-threatening reaction that often starts with swelling around the mouth and throat, but also affects the whole body. It can be fatal if not treated urgently with orthodox medicine. Peanut allergy is the condition that most often hits the headlines, but anaphylaxis can occur with other foods (such as shellfish) and also has other causes. Any swelling around your mouth after eating, or a serious reaction to an insect bite or sting, merits a consultation with your doctor.

Food intolerance

Food intolerance is a more controversial subject than food allergy. The symptoms include a rapid heartbeat or sudden exhaustion after eating, painful joints and digestive discomfort, and generally feeling unwell. Many people refer to these reactions as "allergies," but doctors usually disagree because the underlying causes remain unknown, and may not even involve the immune system.

Food intolerance often results from foods that are eaten every day, such as wheat and cow's milk. Finding alternatives to these common foods for two or three days each week may help to reduce the risk of developing intolerance. For example, wheat can be replaced by rye, barley, rice, corn, or other sources of starch, such as beans or root vegetables. Cow's milk can be replaced with soy or nut milks, or milk from another animal such as a goat. Many people find that the foods that upset them change over time and it is often possible to reintroduce the offending foods after they have been excluded for a while. However, it is best then to avoid eating these more often than twice a week.

Excluding a wide range of suspect foods from the diet can cause nutritional deficiencies and, sadly, there have been some deaths from malnutrition when a strict exclusion diet has been followed unwisely. It is, therefore, essential before changing your diet to seek guidance from a qualified health professional with a special interest in allergic illnesses, especially if you seem to be intolerant of several foods. Doctors who practice environmental medicine recommend minimizing the risk of developing food intolerance by eating fresh food in season and eating as wide a range of different foods as possible.

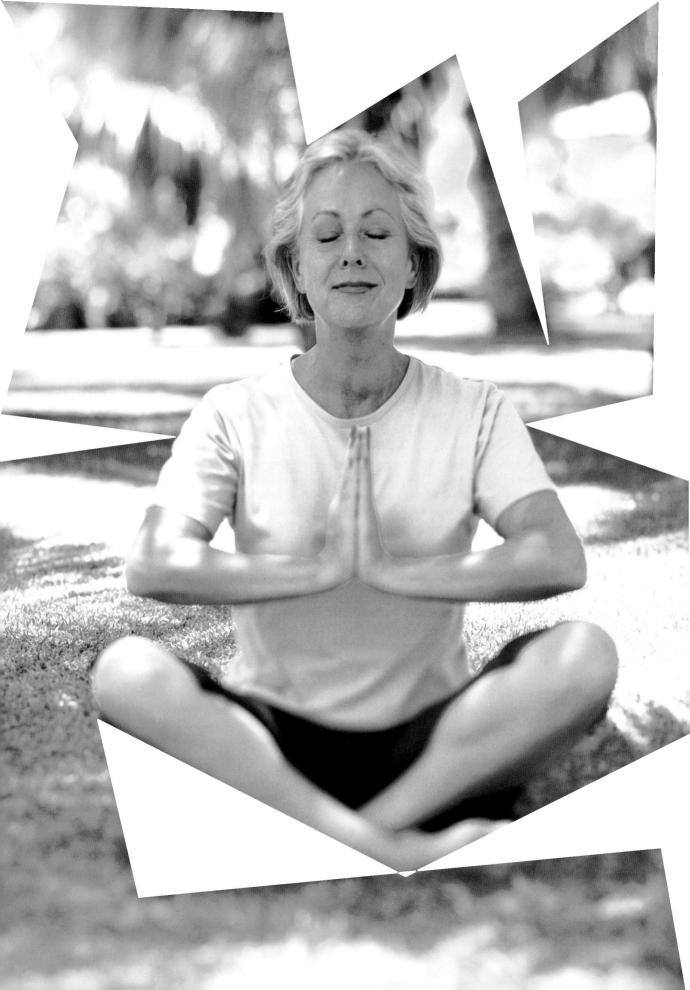

Chapter Four

LIFESTYLE
CHANGES

How you feel influences how you look. A positive approach to life and good health radiate through your face and behavior. At 50+ you may have lost your youth, but a mature appearance can be no less attractive – and is only enhanced by the wisdom gained from living.

"This is how fifty looks now."

The writer Gloria Steinem on being told by a journalist that she did not look her age.

THE WISDOM YEARS

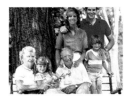

Members of the baby-boomer generation, born after the Second World War, are now in their fifties. During their lives they have experienced radical changes in behavior, attitudes, and fashion, and many of them are more ambitious than their predecessors were at 50+. Actor Jack Nicholson at 55 said, "Our parents' generation was ancient at our age, past it. We are more active, [we] take care of ourselves. We're the new old."

For many people, being 50+ can be the best time of their lives. Life expectancy is increasing, and there is less likelihood of becoming disabled.

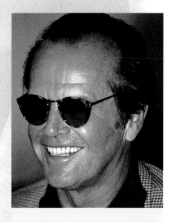

"We're the new old..."

Between 1980 and 1994, the level of disability in Americans of 65+ dropped by 15 percent, according to the Duke University for Demographic Studies. In the United States and Canada there is now legislation against age discrimination. In the United Kingdom, for example, some firms are actively recruiting older workers because they find them more reliable.

There is also now a wider choice of what to do at 50+. Finances are often less strained as children become independent and mortgages are nearly or completely paid off. More recreational and educational pursuits are available than there were for previous generations, and for many people there is a greater choice about the best age to retire.

Despite all these beneficial changes, it is not easy to shake off outdated ideas about growing old. This is partly because, at 50+, most people think back to what life was like for their grandparents' generation. Today many people who are over 70 are living far more active lives than their parents did at the same age, and the majority of people in their 60s and 70s are happy, contented, active, and fit. All the same, it is still common for old people to be categorized as lonely and poor. Some are, but loneliness and poverty can happen at any age.

There is also a persistent belief that a midlife crisis is inevitable at 50+. In fact, such crises are not particularly common and are far more likely to afflict people who have previously had to deal with emotional turmoil earlier in their lives. People who are naturally optimistic are less likely to undergo these crises, but optimism can be acquired, even if it is for the first time (see page 94).

Aging and becoming old are not the same thing

We have no control over the passage of time. Each year we mark the day when we change the number that describes our age. In childhood, increasing age was a positive thing: birthdays marked steps toward independence, the first job, the first love affair, and the first everything else.

We can truly be said to be old when life is no longer perceived as a journey into new territory. Loss of interest in living, belief that things can no longer be changed or that too much is changing, the feeling that life does not matter and that nothing exciting can ever happen again are signs of becoming old. However, they can also be signs of depression (see page 94) and, like any illness, this should be treated.

Even though there may be some decline in physical and mental capabilities, the people who are the least "old" at 80+ are full of plans, and as involved as ever in whatever aspect of life interests them, whether this is socializing with friends, politics, the arts, or advances in science. The goals they set themselves may have changed, but they continue to make commitments to themselves and to others.

Many companies recruit older workers because they are considered more reliable than younger employees.

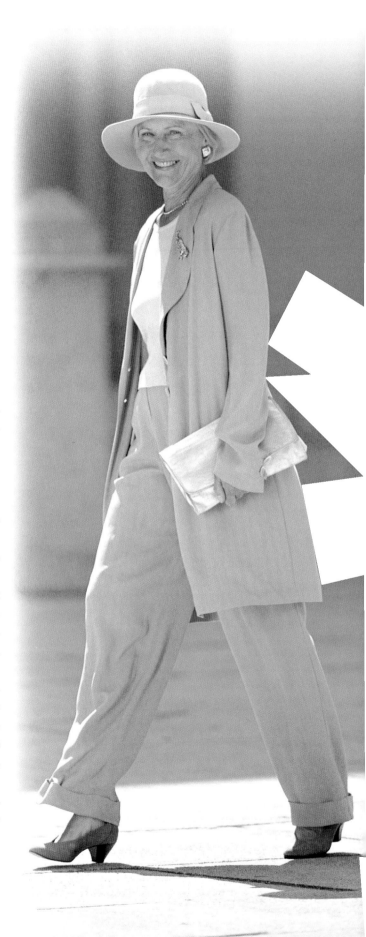

PLANNING FOR
RETIREMENT

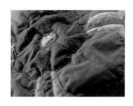

The first comprehensive social security legislation was introduced by the German chancellor, Otto von Bismarck, in 1884. It included insurance against accidents, sickness, and old age. The proposed retirement age was 65. However, at that time life expectancy was only 37 years, and so few people were able to benefit from retirement, even if they wanted to.

Today, although life expectancy has increased dramatically, there is a move away from the idea that everyone should retire at a predetermined age. There are people still working full-time at 80+, but others in their 50s, who are still fit and well, are faced with being laid off or are forced into early retirement. Unless they can find other suitably remunerative jobs, this reduces their ability to provide for their later years.

Ideally, of course, planning for your retirement should start well before the age of 50+, but the increase in life expectancy means that many pension plans that were originated 10 or 20 years earlier are now likely to prove inadequate. Many of those who are fortunate enough to still be employed should therefore seek to pay more into their pension fund and delay drawing on it. This is particularly important for many of the baby-boomer generation who have lived through relatively prosperous times and who do not wish to have to change their lifestyles. But others may feel the time has come to live more simply and economically.

Money is important, but so is the need to avoid becoming "old" too early. An increasing number of people are saying "never retire." This, of course, does not mean that you should continue with the daily grind of commuting to an unfulfilling job when there is no financial need to do so. Retirement may be an opportunity for a total change of direction. This can include working part-time, doing volunteer work, taking up a half-forgotten educational challenge, or fulfilling ambitions that have been set aside in the face of commitments to work, financial stresses, parenting, or coping with the problems of divorce.

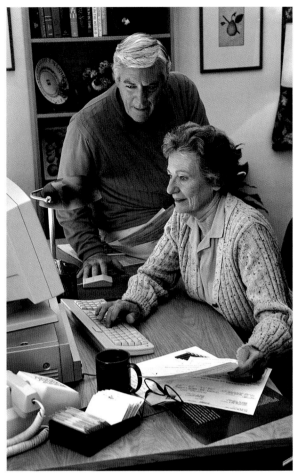

Learn to navigate your way around the World Wide Web, and keep in touch with your grandchildren via email.

New-look enterprises

Find a way to use your skills: as an older person you have much skill and experience to offer. You may choose to apply these in a formal position, such as a part-time consultancy or volunteer work. You could even start a new business, or join (or start) a scheme in which skills and expertise are bartered rather than bought. If home life has been your strength, there are young parents who would appreciate your experience of rearing children or the prospect of "borrowing" a grandparent. Traditional craft skills, such as sewing, knitting, woodwork, or gardening, can be put to good use in many ways.

Learn new skills: you may have missed out on a college education, or simply studied the wrong subjects. Now could be a good time to fulfill those educational ambitions that had to be set aside. Learning does not have to be academic, try:

- Becoming computer literate, learning to navigate your way around the World Wide Web, keeping in touch with your grandchildren by email. Find a 50+ class if you feel that you learn more slowly than younger people do.

- Going to men-only cooking classes or women-only financial management classes.

- Learning self-defense.

- Taking up a craft or hobby, such as book binding, painting, or needlework, or learning to play a musical instrument etc.

Traditional crafts such as needlework can be put to good use in many ways.

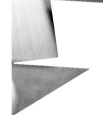

THE STRESS ENIGMA

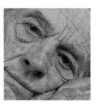

Stress levels are difficult to balance: too much stress can make you ill; too little and you may become "old" in the sense discussed on page 81. Neuroscientists believe that if you overreact to external pressures you are not likely to live as long and may even increase the risk of diseases of the brain and nervous system, including Alzheimer's disease. In addition, if you overreact to stress in your life this can impact your social life, often through fear of behaving in an inappropriate way to stressful situations. A reduction in social contacts can provoke feelings of isolation, depression, and failure, which may impair the immune system function and increase the risk of infection or the development of cancer.

On the other hand, many people think they are stressed when, in fact, they have depression or an anxiety or a sleep disorder. Furthermore, there can be physical causes of stress and anxiety, such as hypo- or hyperthyroidism, anemia, or vitamin B_{12} deficiency. If you feel particularly stressed, you should see a doctor for evaluation and possible treatment.

Reaction to stress

Gauge your stress levels with the following questionnaire:

- Do you have emotional outbursts? Do you feel unreasonably angry or irritable? Are you taken aback by feelings of unexplained hostility?

- Do you often feel overwhelmed, trapped, or helpless? Does your life seem to be out of control?

- Do you rely on "props" to keep going or to relax, such as coffee, alcohol, tobacco, or illicit or prescribed drugs?

- Do you find yourself double-checking that you have completed safety tasks, such as turning off the oven or locking an outside door?

- Do you experience panic attacks, including rapid breathing or palpitations?

- Do you watch too much television as an escape, or spend money on things you don't really need or want? Can you control the amount you eat, whether too much or too little?

■ Is your sleep disturbed? Do you wake with clenched fists or jaw?

■ Do you have problems with concentration or making decisions?

Ideally, you should not have answered too many yes's, but if you have answered all no's, have you just given up on life? Reacting to stress in a way that you are comfortable with will usually include taking steps to learn about and practice relaxation. It can also mean taking charge of your life in ways that reduce the causes of your stress.

Creating inner calm

Because all stress cannot be eliminated, learning to calm the mind and body is an essential way of making stress harmless. A healthy person routinely relaxes by sleeping, by reading a book, by watching an interesting movie, and by getting exercise. Unfortunately, when you over-react to stress you may find that simply keeping still is almost impossible. In this case, you have to deliberately create an inner calm.

Learn to relax. This helps to balance the nervous system so that the sympathetic nervous system, which is designed to respond to danger, is in balance with the parasympathetic nervous system, which is designed to repair the body and maintain normal bodily functions. Relaxation needs regular practice, ideally 5–10 minutes or longer each day. Many techniques are available, including meditation (see page 150), prayer, and self-hypnosis (see page 149), but if you are a beginner you could try breathing from your diaphragm (see page 86).

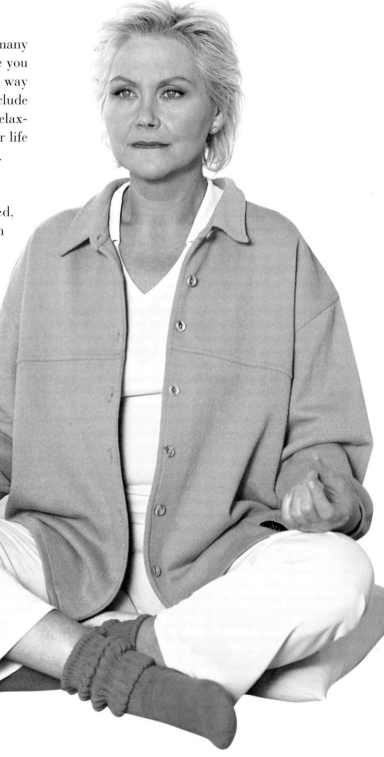

Relax by breathing from your diaphragm

- Sit or lie down somewhere quiet and comfortable, with your feet slightly apart. Place one hand on your chest and one on your abdomen.

- Breathe in through your nose and out through your mouth without raising your shoulders. Notice how your hands are moving.

- After a few breaths empty your lungs without straining, and then breathe in slowly through your nose to a count of four. Keeping your shoulders and chest still, push out your abdomen so that your hand moves out by about an inch (2.5cm). Imagine the air you are breathing in is warm and that this warmth is being carried to all parts of your body.

- Pause for a count of four, and then breathe out through your mouth to a count of four. At the same time, imagine that all your feelings of anxiety and stress are leaving your body with the air you exhale. Allow your abdomen to move back to its original position.

- Repeat the process several times, aiming to feel calmer with each breath. When you are very stressed try this exercise two or three times a day. Do not worry if you do not achieve complete relaxation each time, it will come with practice. The important thing is to keep trying.

Eating for relaxation

Eating regular meals in a relaxed environment can contribute to a feeling of calm. Meals should be based on the Optimum Diet (see page 15), with a limited intake of caffeine and alcohol. Reduce the amount of salt you eat and increase your potassium intake by eating plenty of fresh produce. Avoid sugars and refined carbohydrates since stress can be increased when the level of sugar in the blood is poorly controlled (see page

Adjust the balance between work and relaxation by taking frequent breaks and vacations.

16). You may also be helped by taking steps to reduce food intolerance (see page 77) and irritable bowel symptoms (see page 37).

Take charge of your life

Lifestyle changes can radically reduce the amount of stress that you face each day. This means making choices about your life, about what you want to achieve for yourself and how you can best do this.

- *Take charge of time*: make lists and decide on priorities. Let go of things you cannot control and make positive decisions. Perhaps limit the amount of time you are available to others on the telephone, fax machine, or by email.

- *Adjust your pace*: a sense of hurry left over from a busy life may not need to be continued.

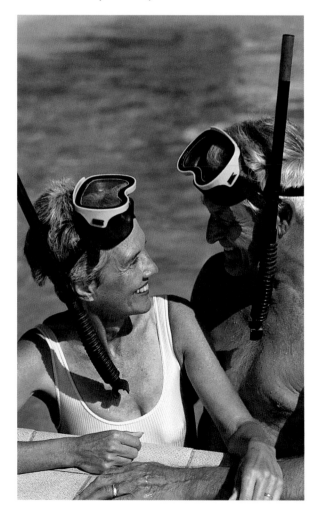

- *Learn from children*: they don't hurry unless it suits them.

- *Consider moving to a smaller house* or apartment if you are not enjoying the time needed to maintain your house and garden.

- *Take frequent breaks*, and adjust the balance between work and recreation. Take time out for music, reading, meditation, sitting and thinking, or communing with nature, and practice relaxation (see opposite page and pages 104–5).

- *Plan regular vacations* and use these to explore new places, even if they are only local and near your home.

- *Get regular exercise* (see page 52): this can greatly reduce muscular tension and often improves sleep (see page 96).

- *Be adaptable*: it is easy to get into a rut. Try new ideas (see Part Two, page 106) or different forms of exercise. Do things for other people.

- *Make a place for laughter* in your life: in India there are clubs where members gather just to laugh. Rent an amusing video or read a comic book. Laughing is one way to lessen pain (see page 104), and it is known to reduce the production of epinephrine, which causes anxiety, and to boost the immune system.

- *Reduce the chemical stimulants* and depressants that you consume, such as coffee, alcohol, tobacco, and other drugs.

- *Share your problems*, and listen to other people's problems, but avoid becoming a bore: if necessary, find a professional listener, such as a counselor (see pages 146–7).

- *Tune into your body*: if your head aches or you feel anxious, try to discover why, and then deal with the cause.

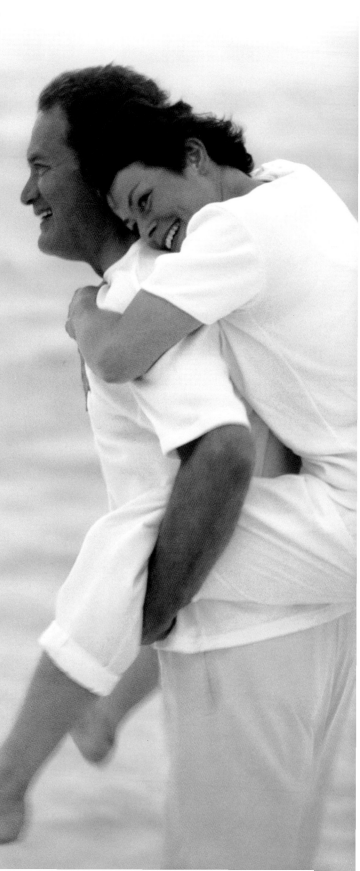

Make a place for laughter in your life.

THE **BRAIN**: **USE** IT OR **LOSE** IT

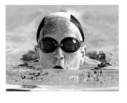

Energy may be in increasingly short supply as we get older. This is entirely natural, but to keep your brain at its peak it is important to try to maintain your skills and interests and even to develop new ones. All the skills you have acquired remain stored in the brain, but retrieving them becomes increasingly difficult the longer they are left untapped. As you learn a skill for the first time, circuits are established in the brain and the ability to perform it is maintained and enhanced with use.

Don't make the mistake of Charles Darwin. He recalled that devotion to his scientific work had prevented him from keeping up his earlier interest in the arts, and he regretted that in old age he could not rekindle this interest. Maintaining skills and interests takes a little time, but through regular practice you can avoid losing them altogether.

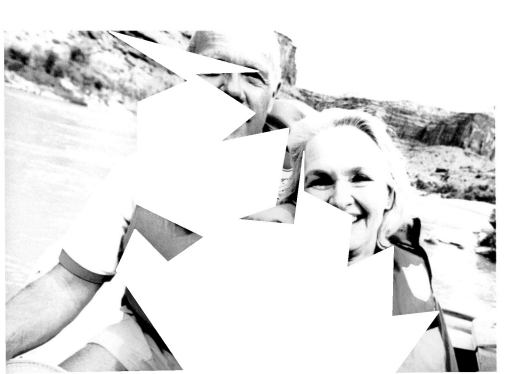

Take some risks in your life and do not be afraid to try new ventures.

Maintaining a sharp mind

- Challenge yourself: don't just accept the editorial opinions of your newspaper – think of reasons why you believe they are misconceived or illogical. Draft a letter to the editor, even if you don't send it.

- Add and subtract mentally, checking with a calculator if you must. Play card games, do crosswords, and play other word games.

- Plan one project at a time: mature minds work better this way.

- Avoid negative criticism, both of yourself and of others. Avoid developing a habitually negative attitude by cultivating ways of encouraging both yourself and other people to look positively at situations and events.

- Avoid striving for impossibly high standards. Try to enjoy what you are doing. Remember, you can derive pleasure from playing a game even if you don't win.

- Seek out new experiences. Make plans to visit new places and make the most of your visit by reading about them in advance. Keep a diary or write an account of your visit later when you get home: rereading it will refresh your memories.

- Long-term friendships can be a great boon at 50+, but it is also very important to make new friends.

- Take some risks. You may fail from time to time, but you will gain from the experience.

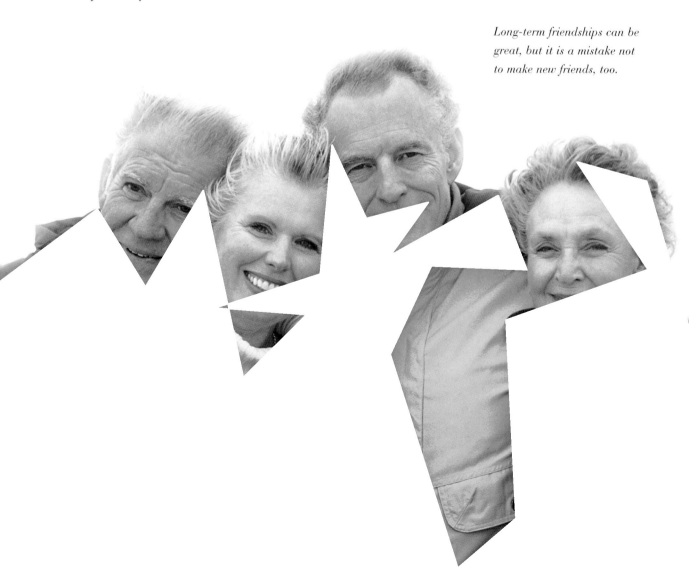

Long-term friendships can be great, but it is a mistake not to make new friends, too.

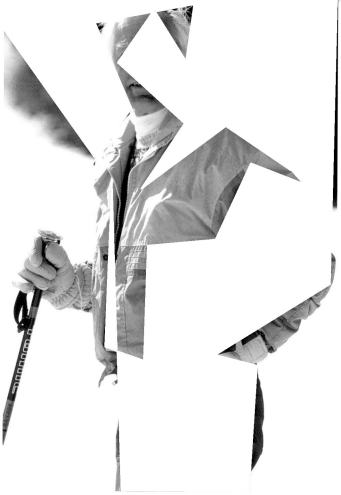

Skiing is a very good form of exercise for you, both physically and mentally.

Learning new things

At 50+ reaction time, memory, learning ability, problem solving, and decision making may slow down. However, this simply reflects the fact that, if your brain is healthy, it processes, stores, and uses information in different ways than it previously did, and this may alter the way you do things. It is known that large numbers of brain cells are lost during a lifetime, but these have been likened to the spare marble that is discarded during the carving of a statue. In the brain, the complex connections between the cells are more important than the existence of large numbers of cells, and these connections thrive on frequent stimulation. At least one scientific study has demonstrated that mental function can improve between the ages of 65 and 75. It is possible that new brain cells, and therefore new connections, may develop in older people: this is known to occur in some animals.

It has also been shown that older people can learn a new language or to play a musical instrument as effectively as younger people. But the way in which material is learned differs. Older brains appear to lump information together in chunks, and this may reflect techniques acquired from previous experience of learning new material. But experience can also be useful in other ways. Another study showed that the speeds at which older typists completed a task were roughly the same as those of young, competent college graduates. However, closer analysis revealed that the typing speeds of the older typists were slower, but that they compensated for this by using some timesaving strategies that they had developed over the years.

Experience yields better judgment

At 50+ decisions may take longer because the brain has a greater body of experience to sort through before a reasonable decision can be made. This same experience of life also leads older people to seek adequate time in which to consider a situation or come to a conclusion rather than trusting blindly that everything will go well. In general, older people are safer drivers, but they can cause hazardous situations if they drive too slowly, and they are more prone to loss of concentration. Older drivers should allow time

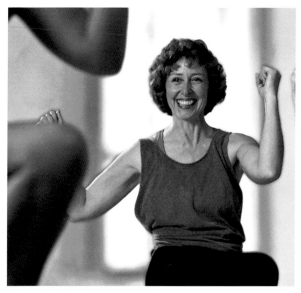

Circulation of blood to the brain may not be as efficient as it once was, but it can be improved with exercise.

for breaks more frequently than when they were younger.

Brains need oxygen

Physical exercise is another way to keep the brain working well. The circulation of blood to the brain may not be as efficient as it once was, but it can be improved with regular exercise (see page 52). Indeed, the physical and mental reaction times in older people who have remained physically active have been measured and shown to be comparable to people many years younger.

Alzheimer's disease

Alzheimer's disease is probably the most feared of all brain diseases. People dread its onset because of the resulting loss of independence and dignity. Families dread the isolation and burden of caring for a loved one who has loss of memory, disorientation, paranoia, and hallucinations.

Can Alzheimer's disease be avoided?

We still know too little about Alzheimer's disease to be able to avert it. However, once you have passed 40 or so, there is little likelihood that you will develop the relatively rare inherited forms of the disease that start at a young age, and there is then little reason to examine your family history with dread.

Here are some simple steps you can take that may reduce the likelihood of developing Alzheimer's disease in later years:

- Get regular physical exercise.

- Take measures to avoid repeated head injury.

- Maintain lifelong learning and mental exercise: these keep the brain connections active and, just possibly, may stimulate the production of more brain cells.

- Take positive measures to manage stress (see page 84).

- Eat well, including plenty of antioxidants (see page 8), such as vitamin E.

- Keep up-to-date with research in medication and alternative therapies. Possible medication includes estrogen and phytoestrogens, ibuprofen, and *Ginkgo biloba*.

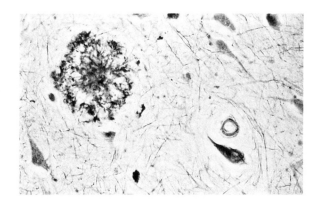

Brain tissue showing Alzheimer's disease.

Ginkgo biloba

The world's oldest tree species, *Ginkgo biloba*, survived the Ice Ages in China, where its leaves have been used in traditional Chinese medicine for nearly 5,000 years. Improved circulation and brain function are included among its medicinal properties. It appears to help prevent and treat Alzheimer's disease, but research is continuing. *Ginkgo biloba* seems to be very safe, but you should consult your doctor before taking it if you are also taking prescribed medication, especially for high blood pressure. An average dose cannot be recommended because each brand has greatly varying concentrations of the active ingredients. Look for products that are standardized to contain 22–27 percent flavone glycosides and 5–7 percent terpene lactones.

EXERCISING YOUR
MEMORY

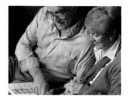

Memory is one aspect of brain function that often becomes less efficient with age. This appears to be partly because the memory holds so much more than in younger years and partly because older people can experience problems in transferring information between short-term memory and long-term memory.

The "memory pill" may be invented one day, but until then your memory can be improved by exercising it regularly. The following exercises may seem tedious, but they can make a real difference.

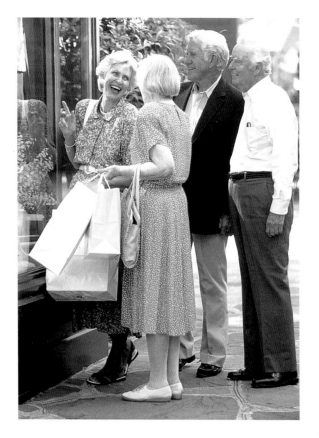

Remembering names

Listen carefully to a name when you are introduced to someone or hear it on the telephone. Repeat the name to yourself several times, leaving an increasingly long gap between each repetition. Try to find a familiar "hook" to fix the name in your memory, so for Bill think of Clinton, or for Margaret think of Thatcher, for Mary, think of quite contrary, for Kirsty think of thirsty. Whenever possible, try to associate each "hook" with a mental image.

Try to create a pattern. This may not always be immediately obvious, but the longer you try, the more likely you are to remember them anyway. Elderly people, in one study, were able to remember up to 40 or more digits after 30 training sessions. Some people remember telephone

When introduced to someone, repeat their name to yourself several times or find a "hook" to fix their name in your memory.

numbers better by grouping them in twos, for example 34, 67, 86 may be easier than 346786.

Remembering what you have read

If you wish to remember something that you have read, think about it for a few minutes, and make a brief mental summary. Think of some questions about the topic and reread the text again, checking the answers against your questions. Use other parts of your brain by talking aloud about the subject, either to yourself or to someone else, and by writing a brief summary. Repeat the exercise a couple of days later, recalling the subject matter from your memory.

Thinking of some questions about the subject is an excellent exercise for boosting your memory.

Losing things and forgetting things

Allocate a place to keep things – like keys – that you use every day. Try to make a habit of putting possessions away in their assigned places. If you change these places, such as after tidying a cupboard or drawer, write a list to remind yourself of the new locations. Whenever you go out or leave someone else's house, make a habit of checking that you have everything you need. When you are shopping, make a mental note of the number of items you are carrying. If you lose something, pause for a minute and try to visualize where or when you last used it.

Make lists

Do not overburden your memory unnecessarily. It is often better to write down a list of what has to be done and check off items as you do them. Add jobs as you think of them. You are likely to

achieve more by doing one thing at a time, unless it is one of those complex tasks that you have done so often that it is recorded in the memory as a single sequence. When you have an idea, or think of something you want to tell someone, write it down.

Every little bit helps...

- Try not to get upset when your memory is having a hiccup. Relax! Given time you will often eventually remember what you had forgotten.

- Always eat breakfast. Breakfast boosts the mental function, especially when it contains some protein and fat.

- Exercise regularly, stand, and sit erect: these help to boost the blood supply to the brain.

ALTERATION OF MOOD: **ANXIETY** AND **DEPRESSION**

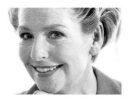

From around 50+, anxiety and persistent negative thoughts about the aging process can be a problem. Fear of aging is contagious and is made worse, particularly for women, by the current emphasis on physical appearance and the cult of youth. These may make you reluctant to go to the movies or restaurants that are popular with younger people. If you experience such problems then there are options. Psychotherapy (see page 146) can be useful for individuals if they think that their unhappiness is due to painful childhood or adult experiences. Cognitive therapy (see page 146), which teaches you to substitute postive thoughts and outlook for negative ones, is a great way to learn how to be optimistic.

Depressive illness

This is less common in the fifth and sixth decades than at other times of life. Depression is not the same as bereavement and grief, which are normal reactions of distress and sorrow resulting from loss of a loved one or a cherished and important aspect of life. In general, these feelings resolve with time (for effective therapies see page 182), but if, as occasionally happens, they persist and result in depression, then professional help should be sought.

Worry

Some people are born worriers while others find that at 50+ they start to worry more than they previously did. A good way to counter this is to think about all the things that you have worried about in the past but which never happened – or if they did happen, how you rose to the occasion and overcame them. Most worrying is unnecessary, and it is important not to waste time and effort over things that you cannot influence or change. Nobel Prize winner Francis Crick has a sign on his desk that says, "I am an old man, and I've seen many problems. Most of them never happened." (See page 182 for possible therapies.)

Grow a little optimism

Unlike stress management (see pages 84–7), which is a way of dealing with problems as they arise, optimism is a more fundamental attitude to life that you may or may not be born with. But, as experts have discovered, optimism can be cultivated and there is plenty of upside to do so: optimists have a better quality of life and live longer, even when they have the same illnesses as pessimists.

Think, speak, and act optimistically

This may seem a bit phony when pessimism is your natural inclination, but if you persist a more optimistic frame of mind will grow because we can influence the way we feel by acting as we would like to feel. In fact, neuroscientists cannot tell the difference in brain activity between people who are genuinely sad and people who make themselves think sad thoughts. If you act optimistically you will find yourself:

- Actively planning the best way to deal with your problems.

- Asking for advice when you need it, and trusting that you will obtain it.

- Getting help if you need it by asking your doctor for a referral to a therapist or for a medication that can make you feel better so you can pursue psychotherapy or cognitive therapy.

- Accepting that something upsetting has happened, rather than denying it.

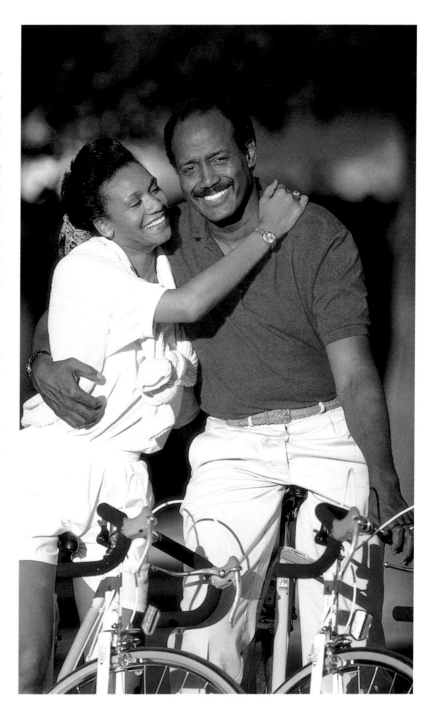

- Trying to learn from distressing experiences.

Try to develop a more optimistic outlook on life.

- Replacing the tendency to worry by saving your energy to deal with real crises as they occur.

Talking to yourself and listening to what you say!

We all talk to ourselves all the time. We anticipate what will happen, or how things will turn out if we take alternative courses of action. It takes a little discipline to monitor these conversations and inject some positive thoughts, such as good advice we may have been given. Even if you have had a bad day, you can always forgive yourself and plan to do better tomorrow rather than bemoaning your failure.

IMPROVING YOUR **SLEEP**

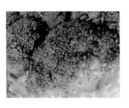

Most young people sleep well: only around 10 percent report regular sleep problems. But with increasing age more people experience sleep disturbances, especially women. The amount of sleep that individuals need can vary greatly: some people require at least eight hours, but other people can do as well with six hours. Scientific studies have shown that the quality of sleep changes with increasing age. Dreams become less frequent and the deep restorative sleep, revealed by slower brain activity, diminishes. In particular the secretion of the hormone melatonin may decline (see box, right).

Physical changes can also be a factor. Bladder weakness, stiff or painful joints, the increased likelihood of disturbance from snoring, either yours or your partner's, all change the quality of sleep. Sleep can also be disturbed throughout life by anxiety and worry, which can be made worse if you start to worry about not sleeping. If you have recently started to take medication and your sleep pattern has changed, you should discuss this with your doctor.

Natural ways to improve sleep

■ After the middle of the afternoon avoid stimulants such as alcohol, tobacco smoke, and caffeine, which is found in tea, coffee, chocolate, carbonated sodas, and certain over-the-counter medicines.

■ Include tryptophan-rich foods (see box) in your evening meal. Tryptophan enhances the production of serotonin in the body, a chemical that induces sleep. Tryptophan is best absorbed from a meal that is richer in carbohydrates than in protein, and its conversion to serotonin requires vitamin B_6 and magnesium, so include bananas, nuts, seeds or green leafy vegetables.

■ Go to bed and get up at regular times, even after a bad night. Wind down slowly before going to bed. Have a warm bath and add a few drops of calming aromatherapy oils (see page 154) to the water or sprinkle some onto your pillow. Use a pillow that contains herbs.

■ If you or your partner snores heavily, talk to your doctor. A few people suffer from sleep apnea, a condition in which breathing stops and which can cause dangerous drowsiness during the daytime. Surgery may cure the problem, as can losing weight if they are carrying extra pounds.

■ Regular exercise can improve the quality of sleep (see Chapter Two, page 50).

■ Use aids that help you sleep. Reading or listening to music or the radio can be valuable, as can autogenic relaxation (see page 105). The white noise tapes that are sold to help to calm babies can improve the sleep of adults as well. If you are disturbed by early sunlight in summer, buy thicker curtains or install a blind or shutters. Use earplugs if you are disturbed by noise.

Foods that provide a good proportion of tryptophan

Alfalfa	Fish	
Beans and bean sprouts	Milk and milk products	
Beef	Nuts	
Beets	Oats	
Broccoli	Spinach	
Brussels sprouts	Turkey	
Cauliflower	Watercress	

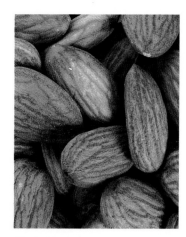

Almonds

Melatonin

Melatonin is a hormone that is secreted by the pineal gland in the brain. Its exact function is poorly understood, but it is known to govern the internal "clock" that regulates the secretion of a number of hormones, and to regulate sleep and wakefulness. The amount of melatonin produced can change with altered day length, which may be the reason why light therapy is beneficial in seasonal affective disorder (SAD). Melatonin supplements may improve the symptoms of jet lag. Chronic use of melatonin can cause depression. Dosage should be from 0.5–3.0mg and taken at bedtime. Government regulation of melatonin supplements varies from country to country. Melatonin is available over-the-counter in the United States, and in Canada it may be imported for personal use, which is defined as a three-month supply.

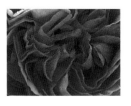

SEX
AT 50+

There are a number of myths associated with sexual activity in later years, and these can cause concern in people whose sexual appetite remains strong. Some beliefs still linger: that sexual performance will decline rapidly after middle age and that the problems associated with aging will, in any case, preclude any interest in sexual activity. In fact, most loving couples are sexually active in their sixties and 20 percent remain active into their eighties: this may escape the attention of the staff of nursing care homes who often discourage any intimacy or privacy.

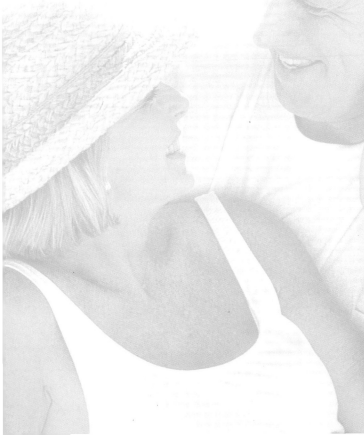

There are changes in sexual performance at 50+, but they are often regarded as blessings: urgency being replaced by calmer, more considered love-making. At 50+ there is often greater privacy, because the children are less frequently at home, and there may also be more time for sex after retirement. Sensual pleasure can become more important than achieving an orgasm. Honest talk about adjusting to changes in your sex life can be valuable, as can reading some books on the subject. However, if you do not have a regular partner, you should continue to practice "safe sex" since AIDS is not confined to young people.

Physical changes

After the age of about 50, it is normal for a man to achieve an erection more slowly, and less frequently. The reason is not clear: it may be the result of lower testosterone levels or due to decreased blood supply to the penis. The erect penis may be less rigid, ejaculation less powerful, and the quantity of semen reduced. Some men choose not to ejaculate every time they make love, and in some cultures this practice is encouraged. When appropriate, your doctor can advise you about the use of Viagra (for erectile dysfunction), injections into the penis, and other aids to achieving and sustaining erections.

Women's needs and desires often change by menopause. Some are liberated by the freedom of not having to worry about contraception, while others lose their sexual desire. Loss of estrogen after the menopause may delay or reduce sexual arousal, and also causes thinning of the lining of the vagina. Vaginal dryness can then become a problem, but normal lubrication will often eventually occur, especially in women who have regular sexual intercourse. If necessary, lubrication with proprietary lubricants or the use of local estrogen creams can be useful.

If your libido is waning...

- Warm baths before sex can help to relax you and also reduce joint stiffness: but some people say that cold baths improve your sex life.

- If anxiety is a problem, try to reduce stress generally (see page 84), or adopt some home therapies, such as massage (see page 120) or aromatherapy (see page 151). Moderate amounts of alcohol can lower inhibition.

- Regular exercise boosts sex hormones. Zinc and vitamin B_6 may help in the production of testosterone. But note that high dosages of vitamin B_6 (above 200mg) can cause peripheral neuropathy; high dosages of zinc (above 40mg per day for men and 32mg for women over six weeks) can impair immune function.

- Medication can alter your libido or sexual performance: your doctor may be able to suggest an alternative treatment.

- Increasing disability can lead to fear of hurting your partner or difficulty in finding a comfortable position. Try different positions – there are plenty of ideas in books – or seek professional counseling; these problems can often be overcome.

Looking and feeling good creates a positive and very desirable image.

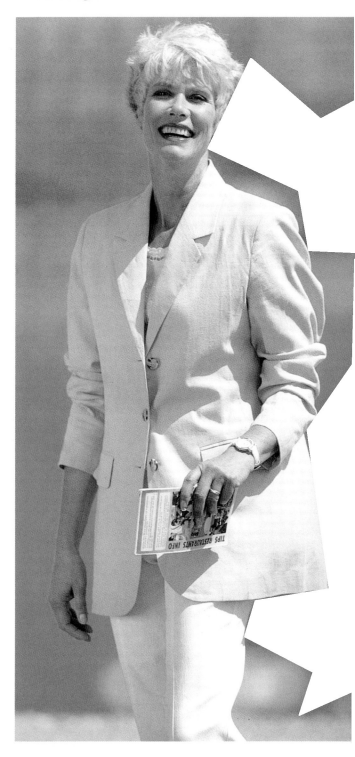

CARING FOR **ELDERLY** RELATIVES

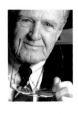

Caring for elderly relatives can be a burden, especially if they are mentally impaired or physically frail, but it can also be rewarding, as it is often a time when past problems and difficulties can be resolved.

Maintaining independence is usually high on the wish list of people in their later years, and many prefer to live alone after their partner has died. This is partly because adapting to another person's or other people's needs and habits becomes more difficult as we age. The choice of independence has to be respected, even when it involves some risk. In fact, choosing suitable accommodation in which to grow old in is a decision that is probably best faced well in advance of the need arising, so that a local network of friends and support can be built up over time.

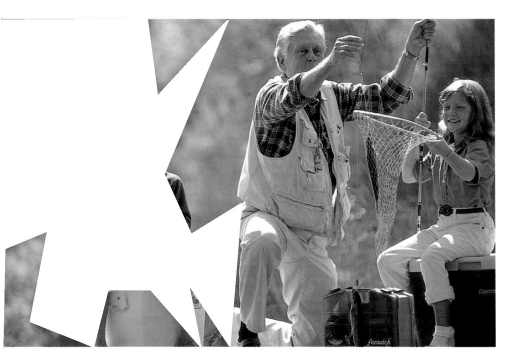

Spending time with their grandchildren gives grandparents a chance to pass on their years of knowledge and experience.

Avoiding isolation

Older people need more stimulation than younger people to keep the brain circuits in good shape (see page 88). Reading and television are both helpful, but human contact is best. One useful rule is to encourage the elderly to have a conversation with at least three people every day: these can, of course, include delivery people, neighbors, or store clerks. However, contact with other people is likely to be more fruitful if it is of longer duration and can include joint interests and shared memories. Providing help with transport is a practical way to help. If you make contact by phone, you may find that making a brief telephone call every day or two to a parent or relative living alone is more beneficial than making a longer call once a week.

Depression

Depression is common among elderly people, and can be difficult to recognize because sadness may be absent. Symptoms are more likely to be loss of appetite, energy, and enthusiasm. If the depressed person also withdraws from society they can appear to be crabby and unreasonable, rather than depressed. In elderly people depression usually results from changes in the chemistry of the brain rather than from psychological causes. This is because after middle age there are fewer cells in the brain producing substances known as neurotransmitters. These are vital chemicals that allow nerve cells to communicate with each other, and loss of the cells that produce them can lead to alteration in mood, including depression. This type of depression usually responds well to conventional antidepressant medication, which can make a considerable contribution to the maintenance of independence. Failure to recognize depression can lead to great suffering and even suicide.

Nutrition

Older people often have small appetites, but they need roughly the same amounts of vitamins and minerals as younger adults. A one-a-day multivitamin and multimineral supplement can ensure that the intake of these is sufficient, but extra iron should be avoided if the diet contains plenty of meat. Adequate protein in the diet is important, as are plenty of water and sufficient fiber. Lunch clubs, shared meals with other people, and taking turns to do the cooking, all help to maintain good nutrition as well as social contacts. If chewing becomes a problem, investing in food blenders and juicers can make food preparation much less labor intensive.

St.-John's-wort *(Hypericum perforatum)*

St.-John's-wort has been used for more than 2,000 years as a folk remedy for depression, sleep disturbances, and to treat various bacterial and viral infections. In recent years, it has been the subject of many clinical trials, and has been found to be an effective treatment for mild to moderate depression. It appears to have relatively few side effects, and this can be useful in the elderly, who are prone to fall if they take medication that causes drowsiness. However, St.-John's-wort heightens your skin's sensitivity to sunlight. If you want to take St.-John's-wort or give it to an elderly person make sure the doctor is aware of your intention because it can react with other medication, especially other antidepressants. Always start with low doses. The recommended dose is 300mg of an extract standardized to contain 0.3 percent hypericin three times a day.

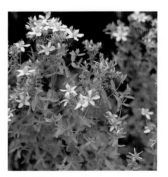

St-John's-wort (Hypericum perforatum)

DEALING WITH LONG-TERM **PAIN**

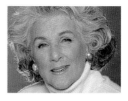

Apart from the rare unfortunate individual whose nervous system lacks the nerve endings that respond to painful stimuli, the experience of pain is universal. Pain is a useful warning that informs the conscious mind that something is wrong within the body and that action is needed. Unfortunately, pain also has a negative side. In chronic conditions, such as spinal degeneration caused by osteoporosis, pain can neither be avoided nor alleviated.

The endurance of chronic pain is exhausting and distressing, but there are measures that may ease the pain and the depression that often accompany it.

The orthodox approach

Most doctors realize that the orthodox approach to chronic pain is often inadequate and can cause side effects. They prescribe painkilling drugs based on their assessment of the severity of the pain and its cause. There are also a number of physical and psychological techniques they can use to help some people, and these should ideally be adopted at the same time as medication.

Assessing the severity of pain in another person is not straightforward. The way individuals experience pain varies. It appears to depend on their genes and upbringing, as well as each person's attitude. Specialized pain clinics have a variety of drugs available that combat different types and degrees of pain. These can be combined with psychological advice – for example, on relaxation techniques (see pages 86 and 104–5) – with other physical methods such as counterirritants (see box, right), and with exercise programs (see page 104). In severe pain, specialized doctors may

also try to disrupt the nerves with surgery or by injecting drugs, or to deaden the pain with a local anesthetic.

Unfortunately, there are side effects to most of the orthodox approaches to pain relief, and these can sometimes be worse than the pain itself. As a result, desperate sufferers turn to alternative and natural therapies that offer pain relief (see Part 2, page 106). But before trying these consult your doctor for a firm diagnosis so any conditions that can be treated are not neglected. Any changes, such as increased pain or pain in new places, should also be discussed with your doctor for the same reason.

Self-help for pain

Be selective with the food you eat: changing the oils you eat may help, but more research is needed in this area. You may need to continue this approach for a few months before you can assess whether or not it is helping to reduce

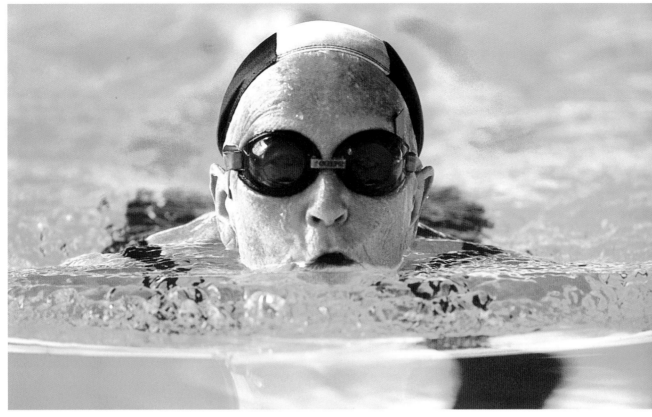

Swimming is a good gentle form of exercise for back and joint pains.

Counterirritants

Many nondrug treatments for pain relief rely on the fact that the pain messages being sent by one set of nerve fibers may be blocked by stimulating other nerve fibers. For example, if you bump into a chair, you can reduce the pain by rubbing the skin; if you sprain an ankle, the pain can be reduced with an ice pack. Why this works is not clear, but the action taken may stimulate the release of natural painkilling substances in the body known as endorphins. Or the relief obtained may be due to other changes in the way that nerves function. A popular Eastern use of counterirritant technique is acupuncture, and in the West, TENS therapy has recently been developed. TENS is short for Transcutaneous Electrical Nerve Stimulation, and pain relief is achieved when a small electric current is passed through the skin in the painful areas.

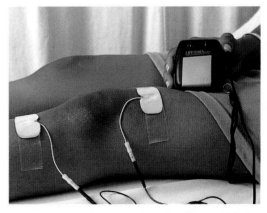

Applying an electric current to the skin can block pain by stimulating nerve endings other than those involved in the pain.

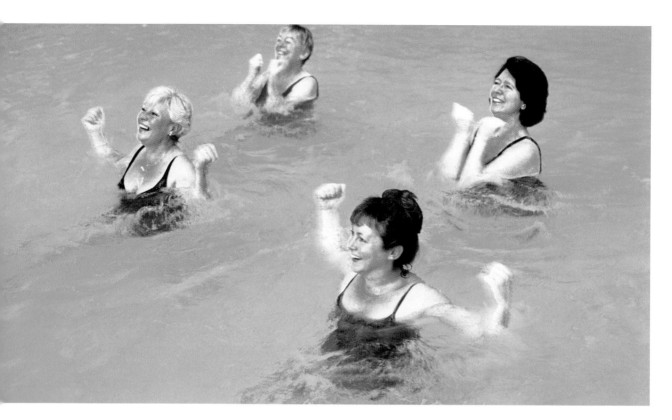

Try aqua aerobics: the water supports your weight and takes the pressure off the joints. It is great fun and a good way to meet new, like-minded people.

your pain. Increasing the amount of oily fish (see page 45) and oils from other plants, especially from linseed (flaxseed) and canola (rapeseed), can counteract the effect of inflammation. Several studies also suggest that using olive oil in cooking or taking supplements of gamma linolenic oil (found in evening primrose, borage, and black currant seed oils) can reduce pain in some people. For other people, avoiding foods that contain higher levels of a type of fat called arachidonic acid (AA) can help. AA is found mainly in kidney, liver, veal, venison, heart, turkey, and eggs. In addition, the action of the natural painkillers, the endorphins, appears to be blocked by certain chemicals in instant coffee, so you should also consider avoiding instant coffee. (See also Eating for Pain-Free Joints, page 44).

Get regular exercise because this decreases sensitivity to pain as well as making you feel better (see Chapter Two, page 50), again probably by increasing the production of endorphins. You may

also sleep better if you feel less depressed, and the muscles and joints appear to repair themselves during the type of deep sleep that can result from exercise.

Reduce the stress in your life because this should reduce muscular tension and the perception of pain. You may be helped by diaphragmatic breathing (see page 86) and autogenic relaxation (see below).

Laugh as much as possible: people have reported feeling considerable pain relief after watching a humorous movie.

Biofeedback and autogenic relaxation
Biofeedback is a technique that allows you to control some of the body's functions of which you are usually unaware. It has been successfully used to treat a variety of pains, including headaches, migraines, arthritis, angina, and long-term pain after an injury. Unfortunately, to apply biofeedback you must be trained by an expert, such as a physical therapist or doctor who specializes in rehabilitation. It is also rather high-tech in that machines are usually used to measure your

response. For example, if you relax while attached to a machine that records the level of your blood pressure, you can see when your blood pressure drops a little, and can learn how to achieve this.

Autogenic relaxation, however, can produce similar results and can be self-taught, although working with a teacher or supervisor is recommended. You will need to practice for 10–15 minutes two or three times a day. Here's how:

- Lie on a mat on the floor or on your bed; it is important to feel comfortable. Close your eyes.

- Focus your attention on your right arm and hand. Say to yourself, "My right arm feels heavy." Repeat this affirmation several times over the next minute or two while you think about your arm sinking into the bed or mat, as it feels heavy and completely relaxed. Do not worry if your attention wanders, just refocus it gently so that you concentrate on your arm. You will find that as you practice you will be able to focus better, and that your arm really will begin to feel very heavy.

- Repeat the same exercise with your left arm and then with each leg in turn.

- Return your attention to your right arm, but this time think about how warm it is. Say to yourself, "My arm is feeling very warm."

- Repeat the same exercise with your left arm and then with each leg in turn.

- Think about your heart, beating calmly and regularly.

- Concentrate on breathing naturally and rhythmically.

- Focus on your abdomen – imagine it to be warm and the muscles relaxed.

- Finally, concentrate on your face, making sure the muscles are relaxed. If you find this difficult, drop your jaw slightly so your teeth are not touching. Imagine your forehead feeling cold and refreshed.

Many people have found that their pain is relieved after a good laugh.

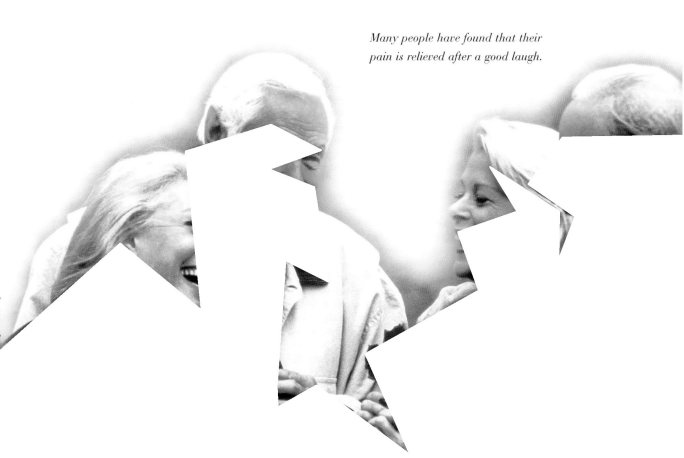

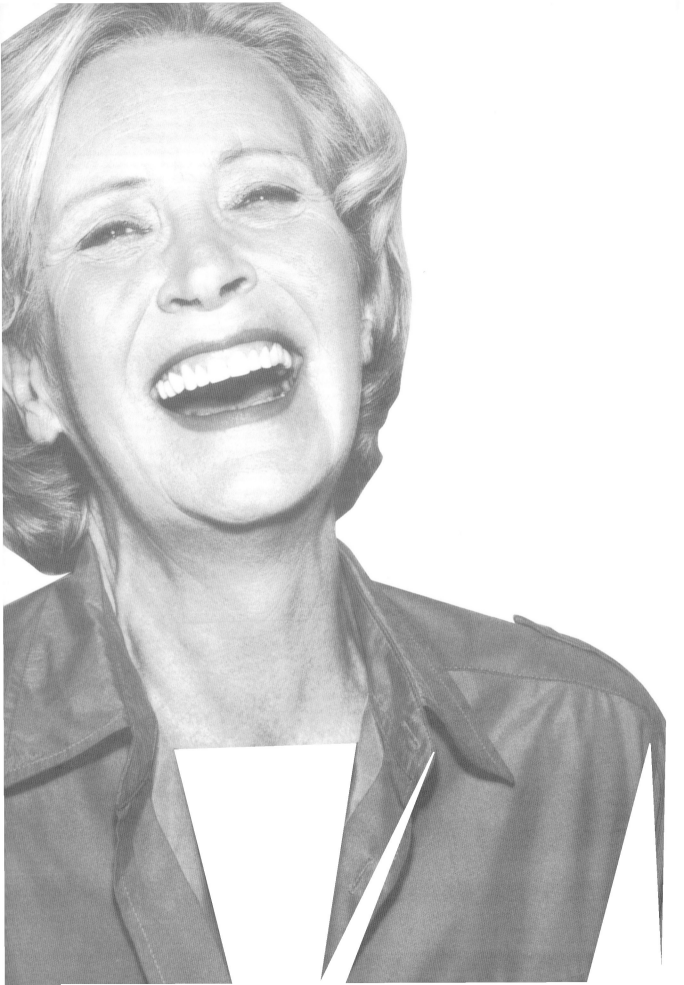

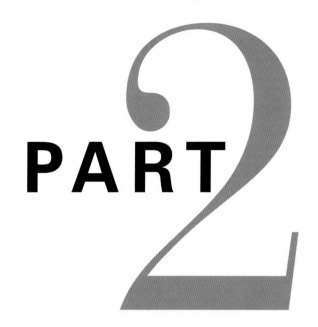

PART 2

COMPLEMENTARY THERAPIES AND LIFE-LONG HEALTH

INTRODUCTION AND
EXPLANATION

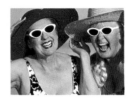

This section of *Natural Health at 50+* contains an introduction to a number of complementary therapies. Many of them are based on the experience, over several thousand years, of finding ways to prevent and combat ill health. When these therapies were originally developed, they were the orthodox treatments of the day. Their holistic approach often includes aspects of religion and philosophy that are usually separated from modern health-care practice. More importantly perhaps, for the purposes of this book, many of them are based on the idea that maintaining health is preferable to having to restore it. Chinese people used to pay their doctors to keep them well: once they fell ill, treatment was free.

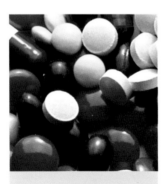

There is an alternative to a "pill for every ill."

As well as aiming to maintain health, complementary therapies are often used for "healing" in the sense of becoming whole and sound, of removing "dis-ease" or a feeling of disorder. They are, therefore, often useful when you are not feeling exactly well, but your doctor is unable to make a conventional diagnosis. It is best to think of them as "complementary" rather than "alternative" paths to health and well-being.

Health care: a new look

Turning away from orthodox Western medicine has become very fashionable, and people often say that they want a more "natural" approach to their problems. In many ways doctors have been at fault. The expanding scientific understanding of how the human body works, what happens if something goes wrong, and how modern drugs and surgical techniques can fix things, has been, and still is, extremely exciting. There is no doubt, to anyone with a sense of history, that modern medical practice has revolutionized the lives of many people. It has given a normal or nearly normal life to many people who would have otherwise died at a young age or have been severely disabled.

Unfortunately, patients began to feel that, as doctors became more reliant on laboratory results and other diagnostic aids, they were no longer really being heard. Doctors were taught less about the immense inner resources for healing that are found within each person, and the "pill for every ill" approach was born. Complementary measures, such as eating a healthy diet, were forgotten as doctors applied their new scientific skills without realizing how imperfect their knowledge was. They often dismissed other therapeutic systems as out-of-date, unscientific, or even dangerous.

The holistic approach

Fortunately, the climate is changing. Optimal health is being recognized as much more than the absence of disease. Improving the quality of life of people who are 50+ is taken more seriously as it is accepted that this may also result in fewer chronic illnesses, or at least that their onset may be postponed. For many chronic illnesses orthodox medicine has little to offer. Maintenance measures offered by complementary therapies, however, are becoming increasingly incorporated into a holistic concept of what health-care at 50+ is about. In addition, orthodox health care has become so expensive that less costly alternatives have an added attraction, providing they are effective.

Furthermore, the prevention of illness is becoming more important politically, and more feasible scientifically.

As a result, many aspects of complementary therapy are currently being scientifically tested in much the same way that modern orthodox treatments are assessed. This is good news; it should allow doctors to make more rational decisions about referring their patients for complementary care. Some traditional herbal medicines are being examined by the pharmaceutical industry both for safety and for efficacy. Hopefully the outcome

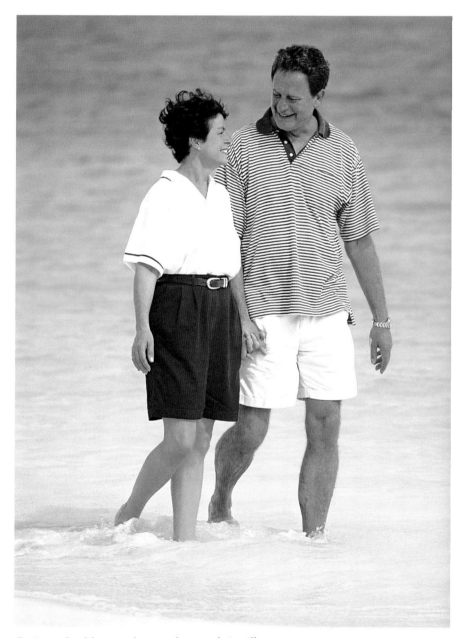

Optimum health is much more than not being ill.

relationship between doctors and their patients is changing to become more of a partnership, with both working together to decide on the most appropriate approach to health-care problems.

Diagnosis

At 50+, staying healthy is undoubtedly preferred over restoring health after developing an illness. However, obtaining a formal diagnosis from a fully qualified health-care professional is essential if you have any symptoms. Normally this means consulting a doctor, who has access to a full range of modern diagnostic procedures. In some states, however, other registered practitioners, such as naturopaths, osteopaths, and acupuncturists, are able to treat those conditions that they have been trained to diagnose competently, and to refer their patients for orthodox medical diagnosis and treatment when this is indicated.

Aspects of safety

Contrary to popular belief, a therapy that is "natural" is not always safe. Just because a medicine has been used for centuries

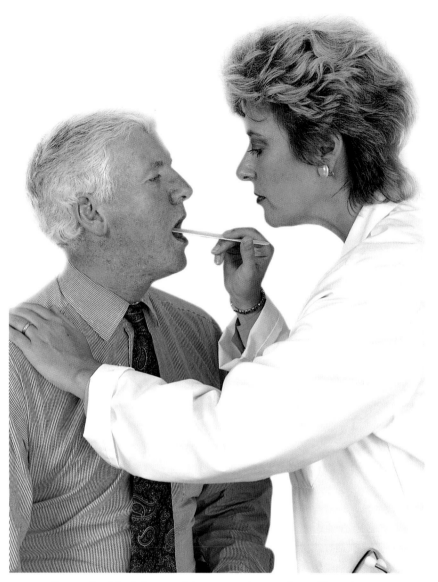

To stay healthy it is essential you consult your doctor if you have any symptoms of illness.

will allow doctors a wider choice of safe medication. Perhaps one of the most exciting changes is the willingness of orthodox doctors to acquire qualifications in various complementary disciplines so that they can provide a wider choice of therapy themselves.

With the greater availability of medical information, especially on the Internet, the public is becoming much more knowledgeable about health and disease. (It is important to bear in mind that anyone can post information on the Internet: what you find there may not be scientifically or medically sound.) As a result, the

does not mean that it is not harmful. A number of traditional herbal medicines have been found to be toxic to the liver, and are no longer available. There are many medicines used in complementary therapies that have not been scrutinized for safety to the same degree that modern drugs and other treatments are examined. Until this is done, it is important to be aware that any side effects and other problems resulting from a complementary therapy should be discussed with your therapist and your doctor at an early stage.

Many complementary therapies are powerful, and it is important to remember that they can mask or change the early symptoms of a more serious illness and may also alter the way that conventional medicines work. When using any complementary therapy, either with a therapist or as a self-help measure, keep your doctor fully informed about what you are doing.

Because this book is for readers of 50+ it does not contain many of the warnings and cautions aimed at people of other ages who want to use complementary therapies. In particular, seek additional advice if you believe the therapies discussed in the book could help children or pregnant women; additional precautions are often needed for them.

Choosing a therapist

It is not easy to achieve a balance between allowing people a wide choice of therapies and introducing regulations about the training and registration of practitioners of therapies that are still poorly understood or researched. Clearly if no one is allowed to practice a therapy it is difficult to assess whether it might be useful. If you choose a therapy for which certified standards for training and professional practice do exist, this should provide an assurance that your therapist has been adequately trained.

Unfortunately, a number of complementary therapies are practiced by people with minimal training and scant knowledge of disease. Legislation varies from country to country, and it is advisable to get local professional advice before consulting non-certified therapists.

Once you have decided on a therapy, arrange a preliminary chat with your therapist. You may find it helpful to ask whether the therapy you have chosen is appropriate for your problem, and also to find out a little about your therapist's experience in treating your particular symptoms. Some estimate of how long the therapy will be needed and how much it will cost can be helpful. This will allow you to reconsider your approach if improvement seems slow in coming.

Diagnostic systems

Complementary therapists use various methods of diagnosis. There is little objective scientific evidence to support the accuracy of the methods below, and they should not be used in place of a full conventional medical diagnosis.

Dowsing is the use of a pendulum to assess the energy centers of the body. The direction of swing (clockwise or counterclockwise) alters in response to specific questions asked by the practitioner. However, to obtain accurate results the practitioner requires good training and total honesty is needed from both the patient and practitioner.

Iridology is the belief that different areas of the eye's iris reflect the health of the body, and that any changes, such as flecks, spots, or streaks, suggest actual or impending disease in the part of the body that is represented in that area.

Vega and similar diagnostic systems use electrical instruments to assess various energy changes that can occur in the body, and reflect its state of health.

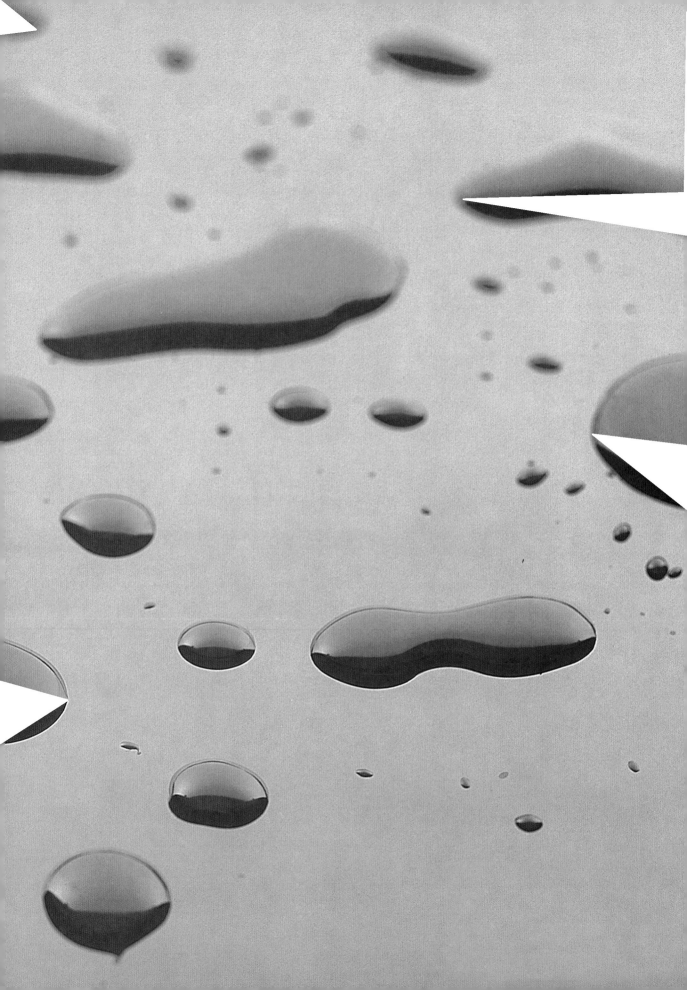

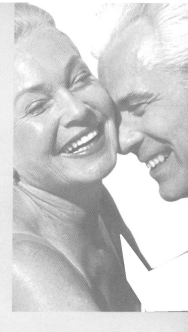

Chapter Five

BODY

Complementary therapies can be used to heal and regain physical health, and in addition many of them can also be used to maintain a physically fit and active body. At 50+, maintenance of health may take a little more effort than in the past, but this is often a worthwhile investment of time and energy.

"Nature is doing her best each moment to make us well."

Henry David Thoreau (1817–62)

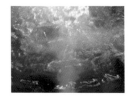

NATUROPATHY

Naturopathy is both a way of life and a therapy. Naturopaths believe that illness is less likely when the body is well looked after, but that problems can occur when waste products and toxins accumulate in the body. The resulting symptoms are caused by the body's attempts to heal itself.

Naturopathic ideas were brought to the United States from Germany in 1892 by Benedict Lust, who had himself been cured by a Father Kneipp, in Germany, through hydrotherapy and the adoption of a hygienic lifestyle. After Kneipp's death in 1897, Lust no longer felt bound by the strict principles of the Kneipp water cure. He qualified as an osteopathic physician and became an American citizen. Lust adopted the term naturopathy in 1902.

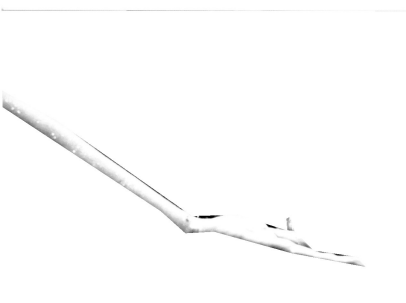

Negatively charged ions occur near waterfalls and are believed to be beneficial for many areas of health.

Modern naturopathic practice

During the twentieth century, the naturopathic movement grew, and today there are colleges of naturopathic medicine in many countries. Students are taught a variety of medical systems that are deemed to be "natural," including hydrotherapy (see page 140) and therapies such as manipulation and physical therapy.

Naturopaths in North America embrace mind–body medicine and often have training in acupuncture, manipulation techniques, herbal and nutritional therapies, and/or homeopathy. A naturopath will choose to specialize in one or several of these modalities. In the United States, a naturopath's scope of practice varies state by state, and most states still do not yet license them.

Naturopaths recognize four categories of natural medicine:

■ Natural substances that are minimally processed: these include nourishing food, clean air and water, and whole herbs.

■ Agents extracted or made from naturally occurring products. These include tinctures and other plant extracts, homeopathic medicines, glandulars (extracts from glands such as the thyroid or liver), and other substances of animal origin.

■ Highly processed medicinal substances that are derived from natural sources and include food extracts, minerals, vitamins, and amino acids.

■ Manufactured medicines that are presumed to be identical to naturally occurring substances. These include hormones and synthetic vitamins. They are less expensive than those in category three and can often be obtained in higher concentrations.

The air as therapy

Naturopaths believe that clean air is essential for health. Exercise (see page 50) and breathing from the diaphragm (see page 86) help to open the chest and ensure that plenty of oxygen enters the body. In addition, naturopaths use various devices to enhance the quality of air in the home:

■ Filters to remove dust and fungal spores that are often airborne.

■ Humidifiers and dehumidifiers to ensure that the amount of water vapor in the air is maintained at an optimum level.

■ Ionizers to regulate the ions (electrically charged particles) in the air. Negatively charged ions occur naturally in mountain air or near waterfalls and are believed to be beneficial for many areas of health. They are preferable to the draining effect that results from the presence of too many positively charged ions.

Colonic detoxification

Colonic irrigation or colonic hydrotherapy has been used by naturopaths to flush toxic waste and slow-moving fecal matter out of the bowel. The procedure differs from an enema in that the flow of water is continuous, and the water and waste are removed from the body through a second tube. The procedure has its risks, however, and you should consult a skilled therapist before using this method of treatment.

In recent years, many naturopathic practitioners have replaced colonic irrigation with the safer and less expensive colonic cleansing, which involves taking fiber supplements, such as psyllium husks, orally.

Because both methods of treatment involve the loss of valuable and naturally occurring beneficial bacteria from the bowel, supplements that contain acidophilus and bifidus are usually prescribed at the same time.

OSTEOPATHY AND CHIROPRACTIC

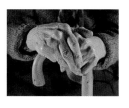

Physical manipulation has been used therapeutically in almost every culture for many centuries: it is depicted in cave drawings that are 5,000 years old. In Europe during the Middle Ages, "bonesetters" used traditional methods of massage and manipulation that were passed on from father to son in the face of opposition from other medical practitioners, such as physicians and surgeons. Indeed, the skills of the bonesetters might have been lost altogether except for Andrew Taylor Still (1828–1917), who developed osteopathy, and Daniel David Palmer (1845–1913), who founded chiropractic.

Today, Still and Palmer's successors receive formal and regulated training in osteopathy, cranial osteopathy, and chiropractic. These therapies are based on the use of the practitioner's hands to treat disorders of the skeleton and muscles, and their value is being increasingly recognized by conventionally trained doctors.

Osteopathy

Andrew Taylor Still was an American doctor who considered that the way medicine was practiced during his lifetime was brutal. Based on his earlier training as an engineer, Still believed that "structure governs function." As a result, he thought that any tension in muscles and joints could place a strain on the well-being of the whole body, and that the underlying causes of these tensions include physical injury, poor posture, and destructive emotions, such as fear. Once the tension is removed, the body has the ability to heal itself.

Today, osteopaths – who are trained medical doctors – believe that human beings, and other animals, function as a whole, and that all their physical, mental, and emotional features are interrelated. Health means that all three are in balance. As a result, adjustments to the physical body can restore health if this balance is disturbed. Osteopathic treatment aims not only to correct any imbalance, but also to maintain health by means of regular checkups to detect any dysfunction and restore balance before any disease occurs.

Osteopaths employ a range of different techniques, depending on their training and specialization. There are osteopathic surgeons, emergency room doctors, and family doctors. Gentle vibration, massage, and various degrees of manipulation are used to mobilize the joints, improve the function of soft tissue, and enhance

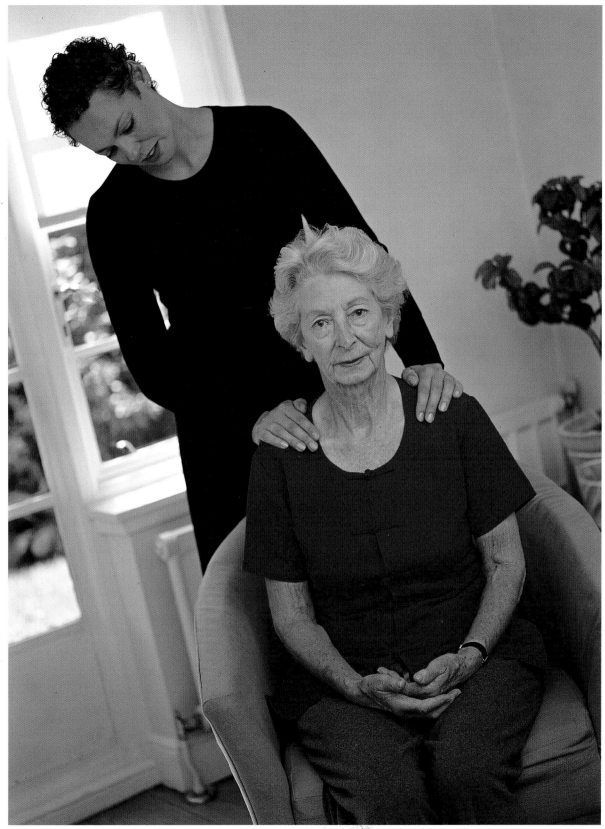

Massage, gentle vibration, and manipulation can all
help improve circulation, movement of the joints, and the
removal of waste products from the body.

Rolfing and Hellerwork

Rolfing focuses on the manipulation of the connective tissue by deep massage, to restore a balanced alignment of the body. Breathing problems, pain in muscles and joints, and problems with posture can all benefit. Avoid this therapy if you have osteoporosis, any inflammation of the skin or joints, an organic disease, such as cancer, or a low pain threshold.

Hellerwork is based on rolfing, but also includes manipulation and attention to the way you move, often by using video feedback. It can be useful in treating headaches, pains affecting muscles and joints, and stress-related conditions.

the circulation by relaxing the muscles. As a result more oxygen and other nutrients are supplied to the tissues and the removal of waste products is more efficient. Throughout treatment, the aim is to treat the whole body rather than just the local area of pain or discomfort.

Chiropractic

Daniel David Palmer founded chiropractic at the end of the nineteenth century. His methods were developed by his son, Bartlet Joshua Palmer, though the relationship between them was stormy. D. D. Palmer believed that any damage to, disease, or misalignment of the bones of the spine affects the health of the rest of the body. In a healthy state, these bones surround and protect the spinal cord itself and provide protection for the nerves that extend from the spinal cord to all parts of the body. In addition, the bones provide the skeletal attachments for many of the major muscles of the body.

The spine, however, is also a flexible structure, and there are many joints between the individual bones. Movement can be restricted by injury, which causes the joints to become less flexible. Symptoms include stiffness and pain, and these are relieved in chiropractic by very precise adjustments to individual vertebrae or to segments of the spine.

The consultation

Both osteopaths and chiropractors will take a careful history of both the current problem and your general health. This will be followed by a physical examination and sometimes also by x-ray examination. Treatment follows if the therapist concludes that osteopathy or chiropractic would be beneficial.

Conditions that can be helped by manipulative treatment include:

- General back pain: including some causes of sciatica (pain along the length of the sciatic nerve that extends from the lower part of the spine and passes down through the buttock, back of the thigh, calf, and into the foot).

- Muscular pain in the neck, shoulder, or upper arm, either from chronic illness or after an injury, including whiplash, when the head and neck are abruptly jerked, often as the result of a traffic accident.

- Joint pain, from sprains and strains, some forms of arthritis and problems with mobility in the jaw joint.

- Headaches and sinus pains.

- Postural and occupational stresses, including repetitive strain injury.

- Some digestive or respiratory disorders, including asthma.

(This list is not intended to be comprehensive. It is best to make a preliminary inquiry about your own condition, or ask your doctor's advice.)

Manipulative therapies should be avoided if you have:

- Any disorder in which the bones are diseased or have been weakened, such as osteoporosis, bone cancer, or a recent fracture.

- Any condition causing severe pressure on the spinal cord, such as a tumor or broken back.

- Any condition in which your joints are severely inflamed such as rheumatoid arthritis.

- Any infection of the spine or spinal cord.

Conditions that can be helped by cranial osteopathy (see box below) include:

- Symptoms that originated from an injury to the head or pelvis, including the after-effects of meningitis.

- Chronic fatigue syndrome, or other conditions in which healing is delayed or inadequate, such as when the immune system is suppressed.

- Headaches, painful sinuses, or reduced mobility of the jaw joint.

- Tinnitus, or recurrent infections of the inner ear.

- Some digestive problems.
(This list is not intended to be comprehensive. It is best to make a preliminary inquiry about your own condition, or ask your doctor's advice.)

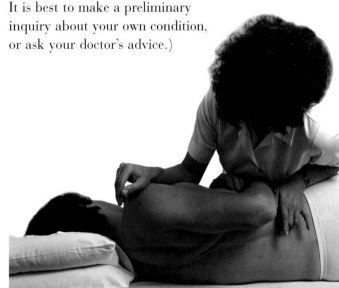

Osteopathy may help to relieve back pain and headaches.

Cranial osteopathy

William Garner Sutherland, an American osteopath, developed **cranial osteopathy** in the 1930s. He observed that the different bones of the skull, which are mobile at birth to allow the delivery of a baby's head through the narrow birth canal, appear to retain some capacity for movement throughout life. This is contrary to conventional thought. He believed that the skull bones move in response to the rhythmic flow of the cerebrospinal fluid that surrounds the brain and spinal cord, and because the bones of the skull can move, the circulation of the fluid may be interrupted.

After experimenting on himself, Sutherland concluded that very gentle manipulation of the skull restores the normal circulation within the skull. Although orthodox medical practitioners dismissed these theories, recent research at Michigan State University suggests there may be some scientific basis to the practice. Cranial osteopathy, when administered by a trained practitioner, is very safe and, because it is so gentle, presents no risk to fragile bones. Although used most frequently on children, cranial osteopathy can benefit people of all ages.

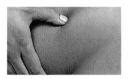

MASSAGE
Every language has a word for massage, and there are written records of its therapeutic use that date back 5,000 years. Massage is recommended in both Chinese and Ayurvedic medical texts. The Greek doctor Hippocrates used friction to treat sprains and dislocations, and kneading to treat constipation. He declared that the physician must be "experienced in many things, but assuredly rubbing." He believed that a scented bath and a massage with oil each day make a vital contribution to health. The Romans introduced massage throughout much of Europe, and it continued to be popular until the more puritanical aspects of Christianity gained dominance. Massage was revived, however, during the Renaissance.

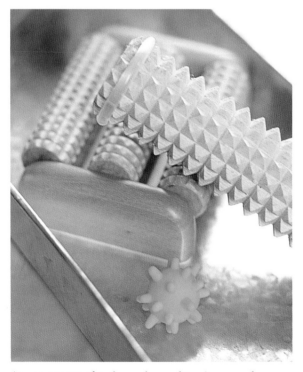

An assortment of tools can be used to give a good, relaxing massage.

Early in the nineteenth century Per Henrik Ling, a Stockholm doctor, devised a system of massage for the treatment of ailments that affect muscles and joints. He created the type of massage now known as Swedish massage. Many of the modern massage techniques used today are based on his teachings.

During the twentieth century a more holistic approach to massage developed. In addition to the treatment of physical ailments, the potential for treating emotional problems was recognized. Now, massage is accepted as a therapy that can promote overall health and balance between mind, body, and spirit. In addition, therapeutic massage has been shown to speed recovery from illnesses, such as a heart attack, and to relieve suffering in certain conditions, such as cancer.

How does massage help?

A general body massage from a friend or partner can improve general health and vitality, especially when given regularly. It is normally safe when used to relieve tension and to promote relaxation at the end of a day, but professional advice is recommended if you wish to use massage to treat specific conditions. A trained massage therapist uses specialized techniques to relieve muscular tension and stiff or aching joints, promote circulation, and help the body to eliminate waste products. As a result, your skin should develop a healthy glow, and the relaxation and pain relief can benefit you mentally and physically.

Massage techniques

The hands are used in a number of different ways during a massage. These include:

- *Light or firm stroking* (effleurage). This is usually performed with the hands close together, the thumbs being about 1 inch (2.5 cm) apart; the action is slow and stroking. This relaxes the muscles and is warming. A brisker action can be used for a more invigorating effect and to improve circulation within the small blood vessels.

- *Compression* (petrissage). Here the fingers and thumbs are used to knead and squeeze the flesh. The massage can be applied lightly, to tone the skin and superficial muscles, or more firmly to treat the deeper muscles, such as those of the hips and thighs. Muscles and tendons are stretched, which reduces tension, and the circulation is improved so the supply of oxygen is increased and the removal of waste products enhanced.

- *Friction*. The pads of the fingers and thumbs or the heels of the hands are used to apply small circular and firm movement. Friction helps to mobilize the muscle fibers and prevent them from sticking together.

- *Percussion* (tapotement). Here the outer edges of the hands are used to tap the skin of the fleshy parts of the body, such as the thighs and buttocks. The movement is brisk, light, and energetic; this technique should only be used for short bursts, and avoided for people with a low pain threshold. It should never be applied over bony areas or where there are broken veins.

- *Knuckling*. Here the hands are formed into loose fists and the middle sections of the knuckles are applied to the shoulders, palms of the hands, and soles of the feet, using small circular movements.

- *Pressuring*. Deep pressure is applied to knotted muscles using the pads of the thumbs and index fingers. The technique is often effective for the muscles around the shoulders and on both sides of the spine.

Myotherapy and the Rosen technique

Myotherapy relieves muscle pain by the application of firm, sustained pressure to small tender areas in muscles (trigger points). Avoid this therapy if you have any organic disease, bruise easily, or are particularly sensitive to pain.

The Rosen technique combines gentle massage and touching with breathing exercises and relaxation. It can ease body tension, withdrawal from addictive substances, circulatory problems, and other chronic conditions, including those associated with aging, such as dementia.

Cautions

Massage should be avoided:

■ During an acute infection or fever.

■ When inflammation of the skin is present.

■ Near open wounds, cuts, or sores.

Professional advice is needed if you have:

■ A heart condition.

■ A circulatory disorder, such as phlebitis, thrombosis, or varicose veins.

Conditions that can be treated by professional therapeutic massage include:

■ Stress-related conditions, including insomnia and anxiety.

■ Circulatory and heart disorders, including high blood pressure.

■ Depression.

■ Pain and tension in muscles and joints, including after sustaining an injury.

■ Back and neck pain.

For the best massage, choose a good-quality vegetable oil, such as sweet almond oil. If you wish, you can add a few drops of an aromatherapy oil as well.

■ Headaches.

(This list is not intended to be comprehensive. It is best to make a preliminary inquiry about your own condition, or ask your doctor's advice.)

A basic massage with a partner

Prepare a firm but comfortable area, such as a mattress, futon, or thick quilt on the floor, in a warm room without bright lighting. The person being massaged will need a pillow for his or her head, and should be undressed. Use one or more large bath towels to cover the areas not being massaged and to prevent the oil from damaging any furnishings. Keep a warm bathrobe or dressing gown handy, for the person being

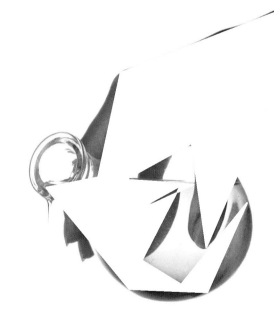

massaged to use afterward. Choose a good-quality vegetable oil, such as sweet almond oil. You can also add one or more aromatherapy oils (see pages 154–5; page 154 for skin testing oils).

When you start the massage, make sure your partner is comfortable, and that the pressure that you are applying is acceptable. You should remain relaxed and keep your hands relaxed. It is better to use the weight of your body to apply pressure when it is needed, rather than tensing the muscles of your hands. Your breathing should remain regular. At the end of the massage leave your partner wrapped up warmly in a towel or bathrobe to relax and enjoy the benefits of massage. (To massage the feet see page 174).

Massaging the back is one of the best ways to promote relaxation.

■ Kneel at your partner's head and use a smooth, stroking movement down the spine, with your thumbs on each side of the spine. Drop your hands to each side and glide back to the shoulders.

■ Repeat several times.

■ Kneel at one side and apply a smooth, stroking, upward movement to the opposite side of your partner's chest, using one hand at a time, and working up and down the body. Repeat from the other side.

■ Kneeling at your partner's side, knead the muscle of the back and shoulder to release deep tension. Repeat from the other side.

■ Stretch the back muscles by applying the backs of your forearms across the back, and moving your arms apart. Lift your arms as they reach the neck and buttocks, and repeat the massage several times.

Massage the legs at the end of a busy day to banish tiredness, but avoid massaging varicose veins. Massage one leg at a time, starting with your partner lying face down.

■ Keeping your partner's trunk covered with a warm towel, kneel to one side of the legs.

■ Knead and squeeze the muscles of the calves and thighs, but be sure to avoid the backs of the knees.

■ Stroke the legs, starting at the ankles, hand over hand to help the blood return to the heart. Repeat several times.

■ Ask your partner to turn over. Knead and squeeze the muscles on the fronts of the thighs, but not the shins. Stroke the whole leg from the ankle, again with an upward motion.

Massage the abdomen with a very gentle action. Kneel at the side of your partner and use the palms of your hands to stroke in a clockwise direction to aid digestion. Do not massage the abdomen after a heavy meal.

Massage the arms by gently stroking and squeezing the muscle of the arm from the wrist to the armpit. Use one hand while supporting the arm with the other hand. Then use your thumbs to massage the palm of your partner's hand using a small circular movement. The pressure usually needs to be firm to avoid causing a tickling sensation.

Massaging the face. Try to find a comfortable position for yourself before you start this massage, so that contact can be maintained continuously, allowing your partner to relax completely. Sit with your legs on each side of your partner's head. If necessary, sit on a cushion and rest back against a chair or the wall. Use the tips of your fingers to perform symmetrical, small, slow circular movements, starting at the chin and working upward. Use your thumbs on the forehead, stroking the skin from the center toward the temples. Finally, return to the chin and apply a gentle pinching action along the edge of the jaw toward each ear.

Self-Massage

You probably massage parts of yourself without thinking. If you feel stiff or tense after concentrating on a task or sitting still, you may relieve the feeling of discomfort by rubbing the aching muscles vigorously. The advantage of self-massage is that you can obtain the beneficial effect at any time without having to wait for your partner or a therapist, but the areas you can reach are obviously limited.

Massage your face

The face has many muscles, which become tense when we concentrate. Relax the muscle of your jaw by dropping your jaw, but keeping your lips gently closed. Use the tips of the fingers of both hands to make small circular movements on the skin of your face. Start at the chin and move upward. Do this slowly to obtain the feeling of relaxation; all the tension in the muscles of your face should melt away. This massage takes only a few minutes and can be done any time, but you may find that you relax more fully if you are able to lie down while you do it.

Massage your hands

For most of us, our hands work hard for much of the day. If you work at a computer keyboard your hands will be doing largely repetitive actions and will benefit from a couple of minutes of massage several times a day:

- Massage between the knuckles, and between the index finger and thumb. Gently squeeze and roll the flesh between the thumb and index or middle fingers of the other hand.

- Roll each finger and thumb between the thumb and index finger of the other hand.

- With the palms of your hands touching each other, interlace your fingers and stretch the tendons of the palms of your hands, separating the palms of your hands and pushing your wrists down. Avoid "cracking" the joints of the fingers.

When you start the massage, ensure that your partner is comfortable and warm.

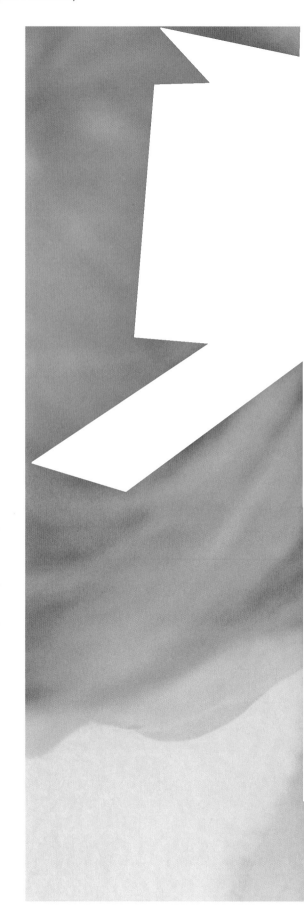

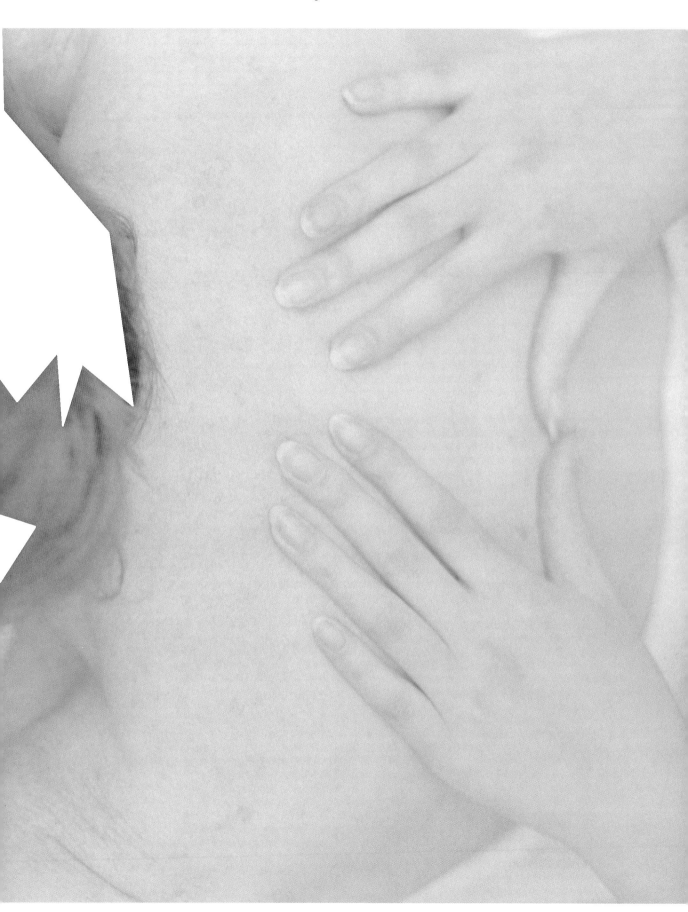

YOGA

The word *yoga* is now well known in the West, where it tends to be regarded as a series of rather slow exercises that increase the flexibility of the body, or as a method of meditation or relaxation. In fact, yoga is a philosophical system in which the ultimate aim is enlightenment, or union, with the Supreme Being. The practice of yoga restores health when it has been lost as a result of psychological disquiet rather than a physical cause, which may be better treated with conventional medicine. There are numerous styles of yoga: Hatha, Viniyoga (meditative in focus), and Ashtanga (aerobic). In choosing an instructor, be sure the style and teacher meet your needs. There are increasing numbers of yoga classes for people with different needs.

Conditions that can be treated with the help of a professional yoga therapist include:

■ Stress and stress-related disorders, including insomnia and sleep disturbance.

■ Anxiety and depression.

■ Fatigue.

■ High blood pressure and other problems of the circulatory system.

■ Pain in the back and neck.

■ Some chronic respiratory illnesses, including asthma and hyperventilation.

■ Irritable bowel syndrome and other problems involving the digestive system.

■ Rheumatic conditions.
(This list is not intended to be comprehensive. It is best to make a preliminary inquiry about your own condition, or ask your doctor's advice.)

Pilates

The **Pilates** method "develops the body uniformly, corrects posture, restores vitality, invigorates the mind and elevates the spirit," according to its inventor, Joseph Pilates. His gentle exercises aid coordination and breath control, while enhancing stamina and relaxation at the same time.

Cautions

Yoga should not be practiced if you have difficulty bending your back, especially if this is the result of an injury. Seek your doctor's advice first if you have any health problems, especially high blood pressure, thrombosis, diabetes, a hernia, or a history of eye problems.

Some simple yoga postures

Simple yoga postures, known as *asanas*, provide a physical benefit. Not only do they tone the muscles and increase flexibility, they are also thought to release the flow of inner energy, which calms the mind. As you practice these postures, you will be stretching your muscles, but you should not strain or feel pain. The positions will become easier with practice and you will be able to stretch farther.

Lateral arc: stand with your arms by your sides, fingers straight, and feet together. Breathe in as you raise your right arm sideways and above your head so that the inner arm touches your head: stretch upward. Breathe out as you bend your trunk to the left, sliding your left hand down the left thigh. Hold this position, breathing normally, then return to the upright position as you take a breath in. Stretch upward again and then lower your arm slowly, breathing out as you do so. Repeat by lifting your left arm and bending to the right.

Hands-to-feet: stand with your feet slightly apart, and breathe in as you lift both arms above your head. Stretch up from the base of your spine. Breathe out as you bend forward slowly to touch the floor on each side of your feet if you can. You may need to bend your knees. Then breathe in as you return to the upright position, with your hands above your head. Gently breathe out as you lower your hands to your sides. Repeat.

Breathing as part of movement

Controlling your breathing is often very difficult at first. It is an integral part of movement in yoga, however, and should ideally be coordinated with the speed of your movement. Except when you are resting, you should breathe through your nose. In general, you should be breathing out as you bend forward, and in as you bend backward. The following two movements are very simple physically, and you can use them to concentrate on your breathing:

- Lie on your stomach, with your feet slightly apart and your hands on each side of your head, palms facing down. As you breathe in, gently lift your head and shoulders, keeping your shoulders relaxed. Pause for a moment, and then breathe out as you return to your starting position. Repeat four to six times.

- Sit with your legs out in front of you, knees slightly bent. Lift your arms above your head as you breathe in, and breathe out as you bend forward. As your head touches your knees make sure that your shoulders are relaxed and rest your hands on the ground. As you breathe in again, return to the sitting position with your arms above your head ready to repeat the movement.

Alexander technique

The **Alexander technique** is based on the principle that poor patterns of body movement interfere with the way the body functions, and can therefore cause illness. The technique involves learning how to improve posture and the ways in which simple everyday movements are performed. The Alexander technique, which is taught by a qualified teacher in one-to-one sessions, can be used to treat anxiety, insomnia, pains in the muscles and joints, and circulatory and digestive disorders.

Salute to the Sun

This series of 12 postures is traditionally performed facing the sun at sunrise and sunset. It is best performed an even number of times, so that the legs are used equally, with 30-second rest periods between each cycle. Finish with a few minutes of relaxation.

1. Stand erect with your feet together. Place the palms of your hands together at the level of your chest with the fingers pointing upward.

2. As you inhale raise your hands above your head reaching backward, with the palms facing upward.

3. As you exhale bend forward as far as you are able, keeping your knees straight. In time you may be able to rest the palms of your hands on the floor beside your feet.

4. As you inhale bend your knees and place the palms of your hands on the floor by your feet (if they are not already there). Take your right leg back as far as you can and rest the knee gently on the floor. Look forward.

5. As you exhale lift your knee from the floor and move your left leg back beside the right leg. Then straighten them so you are supported on your hands and toes.

6. As you inhale place your knees on the floor and move back to rest your buttocks on your heels. Lower your forehead to the floor, then exhale.

7. Without inhaling, move forward so that your knees, chest, and forehead, but not your abdomen, are on the floor. As you inhale push up with your arms, so your hands and toes are once again supporting you, but this time look up so your back is concave.

8. As you exhale push your buttocks up, and make a triangle with the floor, keeping your feet as flat on the floor as possible.

9. As you inhale, bend your knees and rest your buttocks on your heels (as in step 6). Exhale.

10. As you inhale bring your right knee up, and place your right foot between your hands.

11. As you exhale place your left foot beside your right foot, and straighten your legs, keeping your hands as close to the floor as possible.

12. As you inhale, stand erect, and repeat the cycle taking your left leg, not right leg, back as in step 4, then bring in your left knee, not right knee, up first as in step 10.

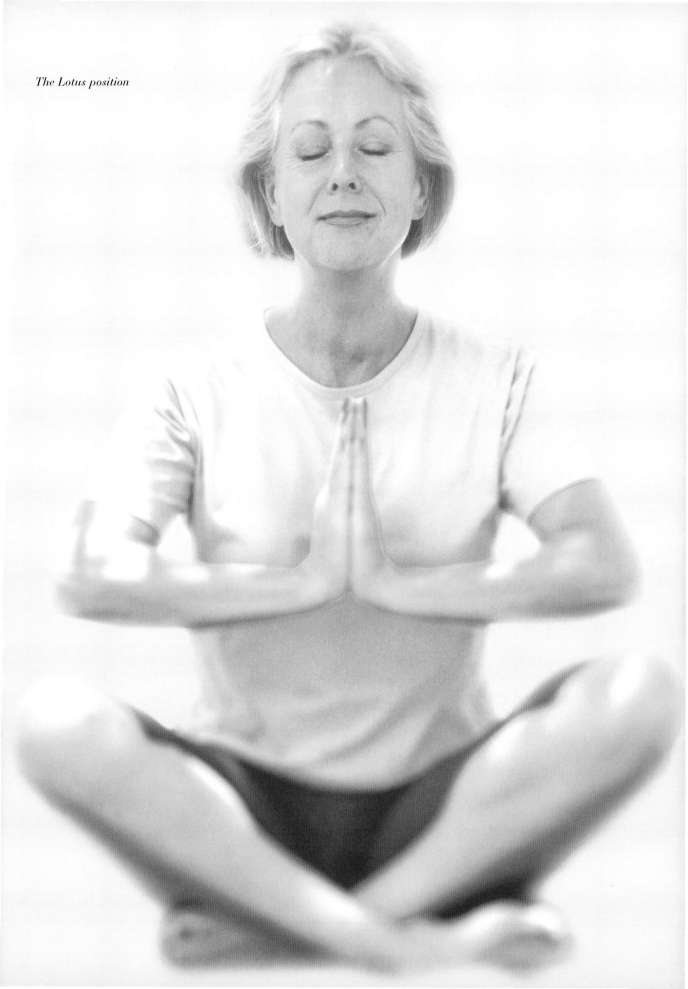

The Lotus position

MEDICINAL PLANTS

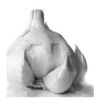

There are records of plants being gathered and used for healing that go back at least 4,000 years, but herbs have almost certainly been used for far longer than this. In many parts of the world herbal medicines are still widely used, but in North American medicine they have largely been replaced by pharmaceuticals. Even so, a number of frequently used drugs, such as aspirin and digoxin, have a chemical composition based on the herbs they replace. In addition, the pharmaceutical industry is actively studying plants with the aim of extracting active ingredients to use in new drugs.

What are herbs?

There is no straightforward definition of a herb. Horticulturists define herbs as plants that die back at the end of the growing season, but many of the plants used medicinally or in the kitchen have woody stems, and are shrubs or even trees. For these purposes, herbs can be broadly defined as plants that have properties which can be used in healing or that impart a flavor or perfume that is pleasing. Many of the herbs that are gathered and used for flavor or perfume (see Aromatherapy, page 151) also have pharmacological properties.

Medicinal herbalism

Herbs can be used as safe and effective home remedies for minor illnesses, but professional advice is needed to treat more serious and persistent symptoms. Most cultures have practitioners of herbal medicine who make their living from applying the pharmacological properties of

plants, but the availability and quality of professional help today vary greatly from country to country. In some countries, almost anyone can set up as a practitioner with very little training, but in other countries there is strict regulation of both training and professional practice. In certain parts of the world, including some American states, it is illegal to prescribe herbal medicines, even though self-medication is permitted.

How are remedies made?

Remedies are made from different parts of plants, such as flowers, leaves, seeds, roots, sap, resin, fruit, bark, or bulbs. Ideally, these are carefully harvested during the correct season, sometimes according to the weather and time of day. Apart from the sap or resin, the plant parts are dried quickly in a dry, warm, airy place before being stored, away from sunlight, in clean, dry, dark glass or pottery containers with airtight lids. Many plant preparations have to be freshly made, but the dried ingredients should keep for up to 18 months.

One of the simplest herbal remedies is an infusion, which is made in much the same way as tea (see box, page 133). The softer parts of the plant, such as the flowers and leaves, are most suitable for this method of preparation. Woody stems, roots, bark, seeds, and some berries have to be chopped or broken, to release the active ingredients. The plant parts are simmered in water for up to an hour, and the liquid strained through a nylon strainer. This preparation is called a decoction. Syrup is sometimes used to preserve infusions and decoctions. This method can be useful for treating a cough or to disguise any unpleasant taste.

The active ingredients can also be extracted from dried herbs by steeping them in an alcohol and water mix, resulting in a tincture – or in oil, resulting in an infusion. Some herbs are ground into powders to be taken orally, while others can be made into ointments, creams, compresses, or poultices for external application.

Herbs are very versatile, however, and your herbalist or pharmacist may recommend herbs that have been prepared in other ways. These include tonic wines, soothing lotions for skin irritations, skin washes to bathe wounds, pessaries or suppositories, and even juices, which are often expensive since they are made from large quantities of herb.

Getting herbal advice

Your first consultation is likely to take about an hour. Your herbalist will take a full history, which will include:

■ Your current problem, how long you have had it, and which medicine(s) you are taking.

■ Any past medical problems.

■ Your lifestyle, work, and any exposure to environmental hazards.

■ Your emotional state. This can cause illness, have an effect on your illness, or reflect how your illness is affecting you.

■ A physical examination, which is similar to a conventional medical examination.

Conditions that can be treated with the help of a professional herbal therapist include:

■ Digestive problems.

■ Allergies.

■ Joint problems.

■ Blood pressure that is too high or too low.

■ Menopause.

■ Problems with sleep.

■ Skin conditions.

■ Headaches.

■ Urinary infections.
(This list is not intended to be comprehensive. It is best to make a preliminary inquiry about your own condition, or ask your doctor's advice.)

Cautions

Herbal medicines are generally safe and often have fewer side effects than conventional medicines. However, it is important to seek professional advice before taking herbal medicines at the same time as conventional medicines and before giving herbs to children or pregnant women. Elderly people who have lost weight or who are particularly sensitive to medicines may need lower doses than younger people.

Simple self-help

A good way to start using herbal medicines is to make infusions of some of the herbs that are readily available. An infusion is similar to herbal tea, but because it is being taken as a medicine it is important to measure accurately the quantities of herb and water that you are using, to infuse for a consistent length of time, and to take a standard dose. If your symptoms persist seek professional help.

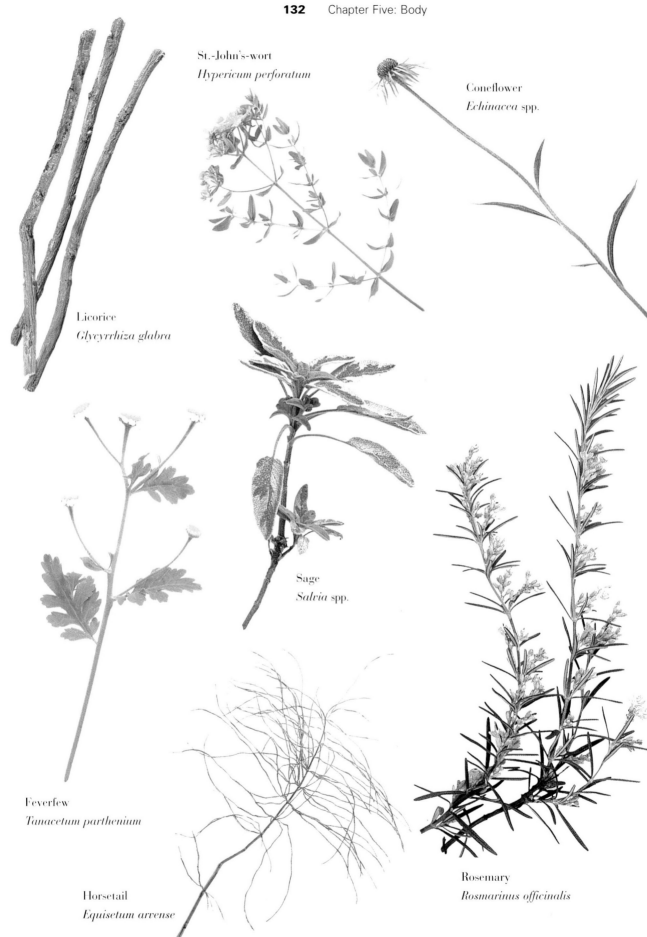

St.-John's-wort
Hypericum perforatum

Coneflower
Echinacea spp.

Licorice
Glycyrrhiza glabra

Sage
Salvia spp.

Feverfew
Tanacetum parthenium

Horsetail
Equisetum arvense

Rosemary
Rosmarinus officinalis

Homemade infusions for everyday use

To make an infusion:

Place the quantity of herb indicated below into a container that has a lid; a clean teapot is ideal.

Add 2 cups (500ml) of almost boiling water.

Infuse for the time suggested below, then strain through a nylon strainer.

Drink $^2/_3$ cup (150ml) of the liquid either warm or cold, up to three times a day, sweetened with a little honey, if desired.

Store any leftover infusion in a sealed container in a cool place.

Recipes

Fennel

What to use: Dried seeds; 1oz (30g), infused for 10 minutes

When to use: After meals to relieve indigestion and gas

Mint

What to use: Leaves and stems; 1oz (30g) dried, or 3oz (75g) fresh, infused for 10 minutes

When to use: To relieve nausea, indigestion, or nervous exhaustion

Caution: Mint can irritate the lining of the mouth

Rosemary

What to use: Leaves and stems; 3oz (75g) fresh or 1oz (30g) dried, infused for 10 minutes

When to use: To relieve exhaustion, colds, the flu, or rheumatic pains

Raspberry

What to use: Leaves; 3oz (75g) fresh or 1oz (30g) dried, infused for 10 minutes

When to use: As a gargle or mouthwash to soothe a sore throat or canker sore.

Caution: Should be avoided during pregnancy

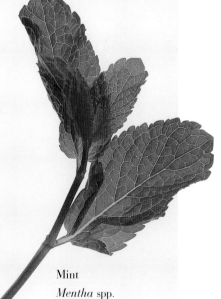

Mint
Mentha spp.

Frequently used herbs

The medicinal effects of some of the more popular herbs are described here. These herbs are available in capsule or pill form, but some of them are also used in the kitchen, either fresh or dried. Doses are not given as they can vary and the manufacturer's guidance should be followed, or normal culinary usage employed. If you have any medical condition or take regular medication you should seek professional advice before taking herbal preparations. If you experience any side effects, stop taking the herb and consult your doctor.

Herb	Possible benefits	Notes and cautions
Coneflower *Echinacea* spp	Enhanced immune system; reduced risk from infection.	High doses can cause dizziness and nausea. Avoid if you have multiple sclerosis or an auto-immune disease.
Dandelion *Taraxacum officinale*	Natural diuretic. Liver tonic.	Follow the manufacturer's instructions.
Dong quai *Angelica sinensis*	Control of menopausal symptoms, and blood pressure. Enhances immune system.	Essential oil can cause the skin to be sensitive to the sun.
Feverfew *Tanacetum parthenium*	Prevention and treatment of migraine.	The leaves may cause mouth ulcers.
Garlic *Allium sativum*	May reduce risk of infection, cancer, or heart disease. Digestive aid.	Can irritate mouth and digestive tract, and interact with anti-coagulant drugs.
Ginger *Zingiber officinale*	For nausea and sickness. A digestive aid. Relief of arthritis.	Avoid high doses if you have a stomach ulcer.
Horsetail *Equisetum arvense*	Stronger and healthier nails, bones, skin, and hair. Control of heavy periods.	Follow the manufacturer's instructions.

Herb	Possible benefits	Notes and cautions
Licorice *Glycyrrhiza glabra*	Relief of arthritis. Healing effect on stomach ulcers and upper-respiratory tract inflammations.	Avoid if you have high blood pressure, or are taking medication for it.
Milk thistle *Silybum marianum*	As a liver tonic. May reduce psoriasis.	Avoid alcohol-based extracts in liver disease.
Sage *Salvia* spp	Digestive aid and liver tonic. Relief from night sweats.	Avoid if you have epilepsy.
Saw palmetto *Serenoa repens*	Relief of prostate symptoms.	Check first with your doctor for correct diagnosis.
Siberian ginseng *Eleutherococcus senticosus*	Relief of insomnia, and from effects of stress.	Can overstimulate in high doses taken over a period of time.
St.-John's-wort *Hypericum perforatum*	For mild depression. Action against viral infections.	Can cause the skin to be sensitive to the sun and interacts with many prescription medications.[1]
Valerian *Valeriana officinalis*	Relief of insomnia and anxiety.	Avoid driving or using machinery. Do not exceed recommended dose.

1 Seek professional consultation before beginning this herb for mild to moderate depression.

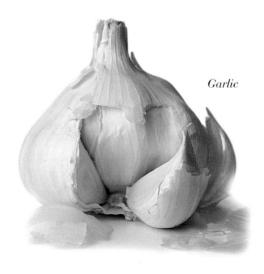

Garlic

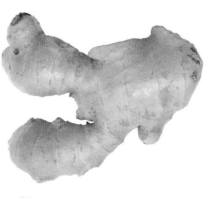

Ginger

NUTRITIONAL
THERAPY

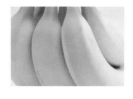

The importance of what we eat has been underrated by conventional Western practitioners. This is gradually changing, since advances in our knowledge of biochemistry are affirming Hippocrates' frequently quoted dictum, "Let your food be your medicine and let your medicine be your food." Many complementary therapists include dietary advice as an essential part of their treatment, but in some cases the scientific evidence to support their advice is inadequate, especially in the treatment of food intolerance (see pages 37 and 77). Some of the current recommendations about what is thought to constitute a healthy diet in various circumstances are discussed in the first part of this book.

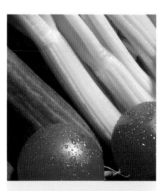

"Let your food be your medicine ..."

Nutrition as therapy

Nutritional medicine is the use of nutritional means to treat illness, rather than just to prevent it or to maintain health. As a science, nutritional medicine is in its infancy, but registered dietitians and some complementary therapists who are knowledgeable about nutrition now recommend certain foods for certain conditions. In addition, an increasing number of doctors are studying and using nutritional medicine in everyday practice.

In addition to fasting (see page 138) and dietary changes, many therapists suggest taking mineral and vitamin supplements. Doses in excess of those listed as the recommended daily intake (see pages 27 and 31) are sometimes used, although this approach remains controversial, except in certain defined diseases. In any case, the use of dietary supplements is never an alternative to eating a nutritious diet, such as the Optimum Diet (see page 15).

The recommended daily intakes have been calculated to meet the needs of "virtually all healthy

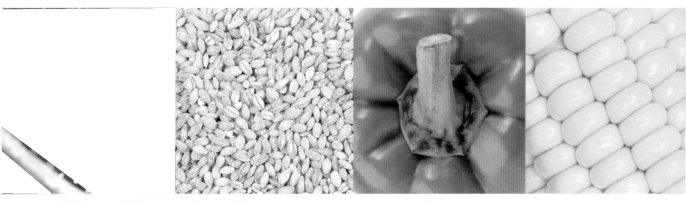

Fresh fruit,cereals, legumes, and vegetables are important for a well-balanced diet.

people," but it is known that needs change during illness. In addition, some scientists challenge the basis on which the recommended daily intakes have been drawn up. They have been calculated to prevent disease rather than to promote optimum health. It is possible that further research will result in different recommendations, especially for older people whose digestive systems may be less efficient than those of younger people.

Conditions that can be treated with the help of a knowledgeable therapist include:

■ Stress and stress-related disorders.

■ Joint and bone problems including arthritis and osteoporosis.

■ Circulatory disorders.

■ Menopausal symptoms and prostate problems.

■ Infections.

(This list is not intended to be comprehensive. It is best to make a preliminary inquiry about your own condition, or ask your doctor's advice.)

The macrobiotic diet

The macrobiotic diet, which aims to provide a balance of those foods that will restore the optimum balance between yin and yang (see page 160), and therefore avoid illness, has become very popular in the West. So, for example, a person who needs to be more alert, but lacks energy, might be advised to eat more warming foods, such as fish or bean stews, or root vegetables. These are considered to be yang foods. A person in need of greater calm in stressful situations might be advised to eat more yin or cooling foods, such as salads.

Most macrobiotic foods are available in food stores and supermarkets, but some special oriental foods are also used. Around half of the macrobiotic diet consists of cereal grains. These are eaten whole rather than as flours, breads, or pastas. About a third of the diet consists of vegetables, including beans and sea vegetables, but excludes yams, sweet potatoes, avocados, spinach, and potatoes and other members of the nightshade family such as tomatoes, peppers, and eggplants. Some seeds, nuts, and vegetable oils are included, and pickled foods such as umeboshi plums and daikon radish are eaten at the end of a meal to aid digestion.

The macrobiotic diet has been widely advocated as a healing diet for many conditions, including cancer. It is generally a well-balanced diet, although vitamin B_{12} and calcium may be inadequate, and there are limited amounts of fat. In particular, the macrobiotic diet is low in one of the fats most commonly occurring in meat and animal products, arachidonic acid. As this is needed for cancer cells to thrive, adopting a macrobiotic diet appears to be reasonable for people with cancer, but the diet is low in fresh raw vegetables and fruit, which are also thought to help the body to combat cancer. As yet, there is insufficient scientific support for adopting a macrobiotic diet if you have cancer.

THERAPEUTIC
FASTING

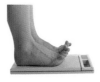

Fasting may be the oldest known therapy. Animals instinctively stop eating when they are ill and most, if not all, religious faiths have a tradition of fasting. Fasting should not, however, be confused with starvation, in which the body has to use essential muscle tissue to supply energy because the fat and carbohydrate (glycogen) stores have been used up.

In its strictest sense, fasting means drinking water, but nothing else, for the duration of the fast. However, many therapists today recommend drinking fruit or vegetable juices to reduce the ill effects of releasing the toxins that are said to accumulate as a consequence of our modern diets and the presence of pollution. These effects, which are sometimes described as withdrawal symptoms, include bad breath, headaches, and digestive upsets.

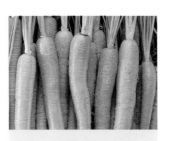

"Pamper
yourself
when
fasting."

Why fast?

Naturopaths believe that fasting is a safe, economical, and effective form of therapy. It cleanses the system, enhances the immune system (see Chapter Three, page 64), improves the regulation of hormone production, and rests the digestive system. Fasting has been used to treat many conditions including:

- Diabetes.

- Obesity.

- Heart disease and circulatory disorders.

- Allergies.

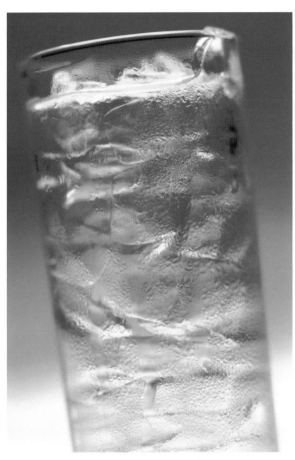

It is essential to drink lots of water while you are fasting to reduce the ill effects of toxins.

- Certain digestive disorders, including irritable bowel syndrome.

- Arthritis.

- Some psychological problems, including depression.

- Skin rashes.

Cautions

Do not attempt fasting without professional supervision if you have any health problems or take any prescribed or regular medication. If you have any doubts about your fitness to fast you should consult a qualified health professional first. It is best to avoid self-medication and mineral and vitamin supplements during your fast.

Self-administered fasts should not last longer than two days; seek professional advice if you wish to fast for longer. Fasts that are planned to last for more than five days are usually conducted in a residential facility. After a supervised fast you will be advised about how to restart eating, but even after a two-day fast this should be undertaken gradually. Begin with raw fruit and vegetables for a couple of light meals, then introduce whole grains. On the second day introduce fish and lean meat, if you are not a vegetarian, and finally add milk and milk products.

Aids to fasting

- For a few days before your fast you should reduce your intake of caffeine, alcohol, and tobacco; this reduces the severity of any withdrawal symptoms.

- During your fast you can pamper yourself.

- Try to get plenty of rest during the day and go to bed early.

- Spend time enjoying the sunshine if you can.

- Limit your exercise to simple stretching exercises and short walks.

- Use some of the yoga exercises (see page 126).

- Hydrotherapy can help with detoxification (see page 140), but if this is not available you may choose to bathe or shower more than once a day if your sweat is offensive.

- Start with a minifast if you have never fasted before and feel daunted at the prospect. Have a light vegetarian meal at about 6 p.m., then have a lazy evening before a warm bath and an early night. Drink plenty of water, herbal tea, and diluted juice, if you want it, during the evening and the next day. Have a snack of raw fruit after about 3 p.m. and in the early evening have a raw salad and brown rice. Have a warm bath and another early night. If this minifast is repeated once a month you can benefit as much as from a longer fast.

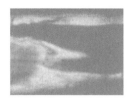

HYDROTHERAPY

Therapeutic bathing is one of the oldest of natural therapies and became particularly popular in Europe during the early nineteenth century. Attempts to verify the scientific basis for hydrotherapy began in 1679, when Sir John Floyer published *The History of Cold Bathing*. These attempts were continued both in Europe and the United States, where J. H. Kellogg published *Rational Hydrotherapy* in 1900. During the twentieth century, hydrotherapy declined in popularity, but it has recently reemerged and the benefits have been described in scientific literature.

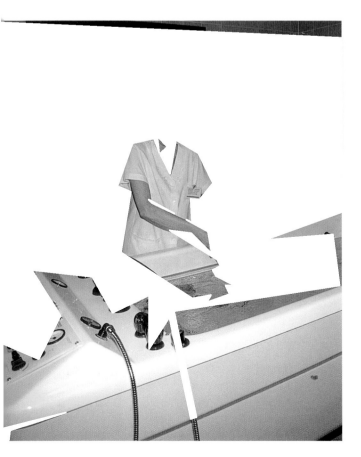

The techniques of hydrotherapy

There are many ways in which water can be used for therapy. It can be applied to the body directly as a local compress, or as a bath or shower. Other techniques include the use of steam and ice. Compresses can be either cold or hot. Single cold compresses consist of a cloth dipped in cold water, to which herbs or salts, such as Epsom salts, can be added. The cloth is wrung out before being applied to the skin, where it will reduce congestion or inflammation by decreasing blood flow. When a double cold compress is used, the cold wet cloth is covered with several layers of dry materials, such as flannel or wool. This has a warming effect because, while it is left in contact with the skin, the body warms the water. Moist heat applied directly to the body by a hot compress relieves pain and promotes blood flow, but it can also be used as a sedative, if the compress is not too hot. Sometimes hot and cold compresses are applied alternately.

The therapeutic effects of a hydrotherapy bath vary according to the temperature of the water that is used.

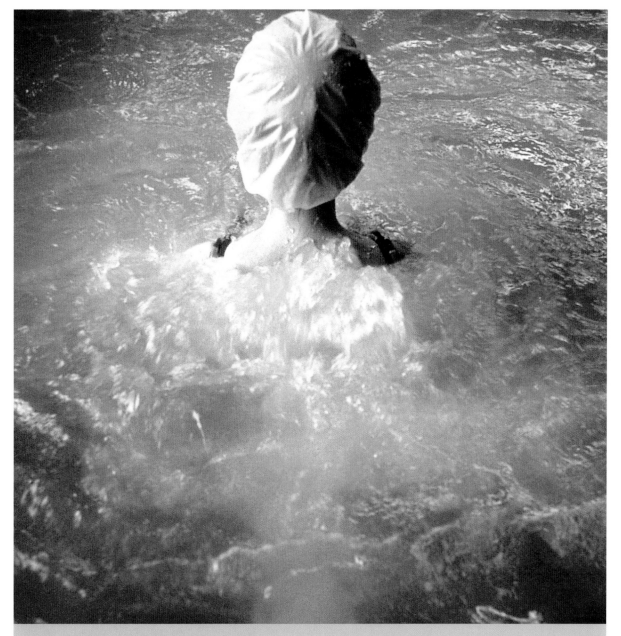

What does water do?

Heat or cold can be applied to the body through water, steam or ice. Methods of application include baths, showers, ice packs, compresses, and steam.

Water dissolves certain forms of medication, so these can then be absorbed through the skin.

Water provides near-weightlessness, aiding exercise for people with inflamed joints or muscle weakness.

Water applies gentle pressure to the immersed body, enhancing venous and lymphatic circulation.

A hydrotherapy bath involves either complete or partial immersion in water that can be of various temperatures, can contain salts, herbs, or medication, and may be still or agitated. Hot baths, in which the body is fully immersed, are used to relieve muscular and joint pain, and to induce sweating, which can enhance detoxification. Neutral baths at around body temperature are used for their calming effect to treat insomnia, anxiety, exhaustion, or chronic pain. They also improve the production of urine and help during detoxification (see also Therapeutic Fasting, page 138).

The sitz bath provides partial immersion of the pelvic region. The hot sitz bath is used to relieve pelvic pain, although it should be avoided during acute inflammation, such as acute cystitis, which is treated in a neutral sitz bath. Warm or neutral baths are usually followed by cold sitz baths, but these can also be used alone to stimulate the pelvic organs, such as for constipation or chronic inflammation of the prostate gland.

The role of the practitioner

Anyone can take a bath or shower, or give one to those who are young, old, or in need of help. However, the unique properties of water (see box, page 141) can be best harnessed for treatment by a trained therapist, who is able to ensure the safe use of this valuable natural resource.

Cautions

You should consult your doctor before having hydrotherapy if you have any health problems, especially diabetes or other circulatory disorders, neurological problems, or are elderly or frail. Unpleasant side effects, either immediately or during the first couple of days after therapy, can include:

■ Headaches and vertigo.

■ Nervousness and palpitations.

■ Aches and pains.

■ Feelings of faintness, or chilliness.

■ Nausea.

■ Problems with sleeping.

Balneotherapy and Peat therapy

Balneotherapy is a form of hydrotherapy in which mineral bathing and the application of mudpacks have been shown to reduce active pain and inflammation in rheumatoid arthritis. Several studies have compared the effects of bathing in water that contains salts taken from the Dead Sea with the effects of adding table salt to a bath. In general, bathing in the salts from the Dead Sea is superior, and this is thought to be the result of the presence of trace minerals, such as zinc and copper.

Peat therapy has been used extensively in Europe for 200 years, but is rarely used in North America. Peat is a unique substance that contains a wide range of chemical constituents thought to have anti-inflammatory, anti-infective, and anticancer properties. It is used in baths and can also be applied to the skin as a hot pack. It is mainly used to treat musculoskeletal disorders, such as injuries and various forms of arthritis, and for some skin conditions.

CLINICAL ECOLOGY

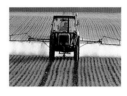

Clinical ecologists treat disorders that they believe arise from an individual's reaction to environmental factors. They are gradually developing methods of diagnosing and treating these conditions, which include allergies, toxic reactions to very small amounts of chemicals, and behavioral problems. Ways to keep your immune system healthy, such as by minimizing your exposure to chemicals (see Chapter Three) and eating the Optimum Diet (see page 15), are discussed throughout this book.

Pesticides and herbicides

Most of the pesticides and herbicides in use today are less toxic than DDT and other chemicals that have been banned, but their use on food crops remains controversial. Residue levels in food are monitored, but only a small sample can be checked. While research shows that very low levels of residue appear to be safe, there is no research that has studied the cumulative and additive effects of these chemicals.

Unfortunately, a number of people have become phobic to the extent that they are failing to eat adequate amounts of fresh produce, which itself generates health risks. Considerable consumer pressure is fostering greater awareness of the problem, which will hopefully lead to changes in farming practice. In the meantime you can reduce your exposure to these chemicals by:

■ Eating organic produce.

■ Reducing your intake of foods in which pesticides collect, such as animal fat.

■ Removing pesticide residues by soaking nonorganic food in water containing a mild additive-free soap or using one of the biodegradable cleansers now available commercially.

■ Peeling the skin or removing the outer leaves of produce. This may, however, remove some nutrients as well.

■ Encouraging your food retailers to use suppliers who restrict or avoid the use of chemical treatments for their crops and animals.

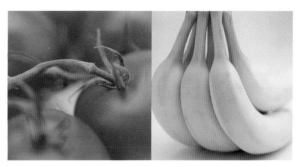

It is best to eat organic produce to cut down on pesticides.

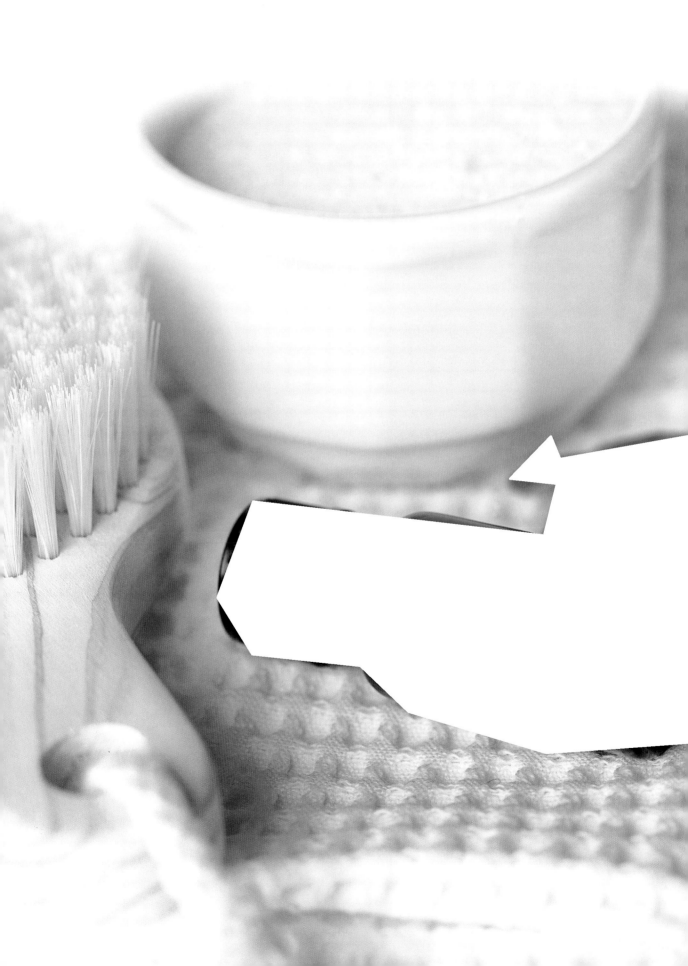

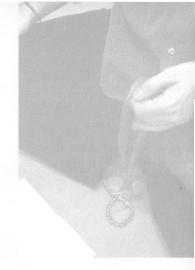

Chapter Six

MIND

Few people travel through life without their mental health being challenged, at least from time to time. Just as we seek healing for physical illness, so it is right to look for help with psychological problems. At 50+, long-standing difficulties stemming from childhood or more recent sorrows all need to be tackled to achieve or maintain the best possible health of mind and spirit.

"I fear I am not in my perfect mind."

King Lear, William Shakespeare (1564–1616)

PSYCHOTHERAPY

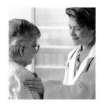

Just talking to another person has probably always been used to heal the mind. Since the late nineteenth century an increasing understanding of the interrelationship between the mind and the body has encouraged the formal adoption of this approach as part of medical practice. Today there are many different ways that psychotherapists try to heal mental illnesses, including depression, anxiety, phobias, and obsessions, simply by talking with their clients.

Some methods of psychotherapy

Analytical therapy seeks to uncover past experiences that have been repressed and subsequently cause psychological symptoms. Once these are recognized, clients are freed from past conflicts and able to build their lives in the present. Unfortunately, the process can take several years and is generally costly. Existential therapy aims to enable people to come to terms with themselves and life as they are. Again, it is costly and requires a long-term commitment.

Behavioral therapy, which is often combined with cognitive therapy, is based on the belief that behavior can be both learned and unlearned, and that mental health can be improved when behavior is changed for the better by learning more appropriate ways to respond to the normal events of life (see box below). Transactional analysis

Cognitive therapy

Cognitive therapy is a form of behavioral therapy that can help people whose psychological ills result from a negative distortion of what is happening in their lives. This black-and-white way of thinking often results from depression, but has its roots in past experiences. Some people learned these unhealthy thought patterns in childhood as a way of dealing with problems at home or at school. When these attitudes persist into adult life, or recur under stress, people avoid situations in which they fear failure, and often give up too easily.

Modern cognitive therapy sets out to provide new ways of thinking about and understanding the origins of the negativity. When the behavior and emotions have been irrational, a more rational approach should be adopted. This often includes encouraging the awareness in clients that they have to take responsibility for their own thoughts and actions.

aims to increase the awareness in clients that they have a choice in the way they relate to others, and in their attitudes toward themselves.

Sometimes psychotherapy takes place in a group. Group techniques include Gestalt therapy, which aims to release the individual from past unfinished business, and psychodrama, in which past conflicts and emotional struggles are acted out.

Choosing a psychotherapist

If you feel that psychotherapy would help you, seek professional guidance about the approach that is within your budget and is suitable for your problem. Getting a referral from a physician or another health care professional might be helpful. Most therapists use more than one method of therapy and prospective clients should ask about which methods the therapist prefers and why. Also, prospective clients should talk with the therapist about anticipated duration of therapy and goals for completion.

Counseling

Counseling is usually undertaken in response to a relatively acute problem, such as following grief or shock, or in making a career decision. Informal counseling was once undertaken by the family pastor, priest, or rabbi, for example, and within an extended network of friends and family. Such outlets are no longer so easily available and counseling has become more formalized. Counselors are trained to listen and to allow space for their clients to review their problems and to understand them better. Once this is achieved it is possible to work out a way of dealing with them. Co-counseling is a technique in which the counselor plays a client role, and the client listens and tries to respond. This is intended to help clients learn more about their own problems by looking at them from a different perspective.

Just talking to another person has probably always been used to heal the mind.

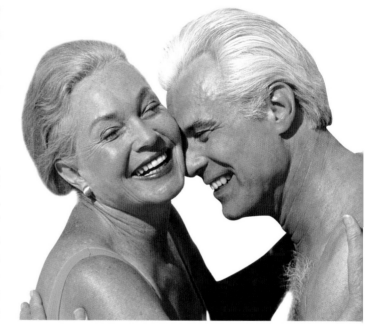

Bioenergetics

Bioenergetics is a form of psychological therapy that is based on the belief that we tense our muscles as a way of protecting ourselves against mental pain and thus avoid exposing ourselves to the memory of past painful experiences. Therapists trained to "read" the way the body moves claim that by observing their clients they can gain an understanding of the underlying causes of both psychological and physical ailments. They believe that helping their clients achieve an awareness of the cause of their problems can bring a release of the pain and the resolution of its causes. This approach can help asthma, migraines, sleep disorders, and digestive problems.

HYPNOTHERAPY

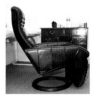

Inducing a trance in a client is an ancient method of healing that has been practiced in many cultures, but it is a therapy that is deeply mistrusted. This is partly because healers who have used hypnosis have often appeared to be in touch with supernatural agencies, and partly because hypnosis connotes something less than hard science to most people. Modern hypnotherapy dates from the eighteenth century, when Anton Mesmer began to experiment with the use of hypnosis as a method of healing. It was not until the second half of the twentieth century, however, that doctors accepted that hypnosis can be useful as a therapy.

What is hypnosis?

Hypnosis can be regarded as a state of profound relaxation, both mental and physical, in which the subject is detached from reality. This state happens to almost everyone when they lose a sense of time, for example, while reading or even walking along a familiar road. The conscious mind drifts off, leaving the subconscious mind in charge of safety. In hypnosis, a person learns how to elicit aid from their own unconscious to produce positive change. Scientific assessment of hypnosis has included the use of electroencephalographs (EEGs) and these have shown that hypnosis seems to lie between being fully alert and asleep. As the trance deepens, the pattern of the EEG changes to one that is nearer to that recorded during sleep.

Creative arts therapies

Creative arts therapies include the use of dance, music, art, and other practical activities to stimulate self-expression. These therapies are based on the belief that emotions and emotional memories are stored in the body and that they can be safely expressed by taking part in the creative arts. In this way the causes of abnormal behavior can be understood. Therapists are also trained to recognize clues that will enable the resolution of the problem by means of psychotherapy. Ailments that may benefit include anxiety, depression, migraines, and digestive problems, as well as disorders of sleep, eating, and addiction. These therapies are safe, but it is essential that you choose a therapist who is registered and holds appropriate qualifications.

Visualization

Visualization is the formation of mental images that have meaning to the person undertaking this therapy. It is usually used in conjunction with relaxation techniques (see pages 104–5) or hypnotherapy. Once the habit of visualizing a relaxing and happy place has been established, the image can easily be recalled during times of stress. However, visualization can also be used to recall incidents in the past, to create images of beneficial lifestyle changes that could be adopted, or to increase a feeling of relaxation by imagining the systems of the body all working in harmony. Visualization can benefit various psychological problems, sleep disorders, and problems with the heart, circulation, and digestion. However, visualization can trigger physical reactions. If you suffer from respiratory problems do not attempt visualization without consulting your doctor first.

Is hypnosis safe?

Contrary to popular belief, the person being hypnotized remains aware of what is going on and is able to terminate the hypnosis at any time. However, even when we are fully conscious we can sometimes be tricked by a persuasive person to do things that are against our best interests and this can happen in hypnosis. For this reason, it is best to avoid being hypnotized by anyone who is not a fully qualified, professional practitioner.

Conditions that can be treated by a professional hypnotherapist include:

■ States of anxiety, such as phobias, panic attacks, and difficulties with relationships.

■ Stress symptoms, such as blushing, impotence, comfort eating, and headaches.

■ Addictions, such as those to alcohol, tobacco, or drugs.

■ Problems with a lack of self-confidence and moods such as sadness and anger.

■ Chronic pain.
(This list is not intended to be comprehensive. It is best to make a preliminary inquiry about your own condition, or ask your doctor's advice.)

Cautions

Hypnotherapy can be practiced by medical doctors, psychologists, licensed clinical social workers, and marriage and family therapists. In some states there are also certified hypnotherapists who are more appropriate for smoking cessation, test taking, and public speaking. A person with a history of epilepsy, or severe emotional, physical, or sexual trauma should only undergo hypnosis with great caution and with a licensed mental health professional. Certified hypnotherapists, however, are not licensed mental health professionals.

How does hypnotherapy help?

A therapist may want to use hypnotherapy to achieve complete relaxation to further analytical therapy, or to implant positive suggestions that link current feelings and problems with events from the past. Positive suggestions can be used to replace negative patterns of thinking and behavior. This may be used to help with problems such as anxiety or smoking. Some therapists induce hypno-anesthesia to control pain, such as during dental treatment.

Is self-hypnosis worth trying?

With practice, a light trance can be achieved by self-hypnosis. If you practice autogenic relaxation (see pages 104–5) you can spend time, once you have achieved complete relaxation, to reinforce suggestions that you want to make for yourself, such as believing that you can stop smoking. You may find a commercial self-hypnosis tape helpful, but it is often better to make your own tape tailored to your own needs. Self-hypnosis should not be practiced when doing any task that requires you to be alert.

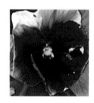

MEDITATION

Many people believe that energy flows through the body, and that illness occurs when the flow is blocked. Meditation is a way of harnessing this inner energy to promote healing and well-being. Meditation forms a part of the practice of most religions, often as part of an associated mystical tradition. However, it can also be a cultural or secular activity, and it is increasingly practiced as people seek retreat to help them cope with the pace of modern life.

Meditation is simply "time out" from the hustle and bustle of daily life. You can learn it from a book or teacher, but ultimately the only way to meditate is to practice it regularly.

Adopt a comfortable position in a quiet place, gently focus your mind, and become still. You may find it helpful to repeat a word or phrase inwardly, or to focus your eyes on a flower or religious object, or to concentrate on your breathing, which should become slower as you relax. If your attention wanders, gently refocus it. Relax your mind and body.

During meditation many of the muscles relax, the breathing slows, and the blood pressure decreases. On returning to activities following meditation, people report decreased anxiety, anger, and other inner tension. Mentally, there is often greater clarity of thought and a release of creativity. Conditions that may respond to meditation include:

- Blood pressure problems and other circulatory disorders.

- Stress and stress-related problems.

- Chronic pain, including muscular pain, headaches, and migraines.

- Respiratory problems, including asthma.

- Problems with sleeping.
(This list is not intended to be comprehensive.)

Transcendental meditation

Transcendental meditation (TM) is based on the idea that you can achieve a state of restful alertness by mentally repeating a short phrase, or mantra. TM lessons are given by trained teachers and should be practiced for 15–20 minutes each day.

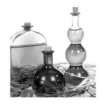

AROMATHERAPY

For many centuries aromatic oils have been extracted from plants and used medicinally, for pleasure, as well as to embalm bodies. The French cosmetic scientist Rene-Maurice Gattefossé first used the word *aromatherapy* in 1937. Although his main interest was cosmetics, Gattefossé realized that the essential oils he was using not only had antiseptic properties, but were also able to relieve pain. He discovered that oils applied to the skin are absorbed into the body and carried around in the blood.

Aromatherapy oils are essential oils extracted from plants.

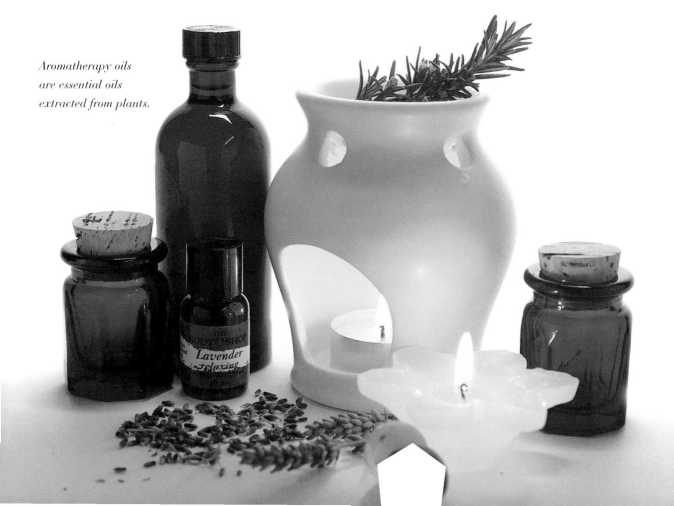

Aroma families

When you start using aromatherapy oils you will find that you have a huge and possibly confusing choice. Some of the more popular oils are listed below. You might like to select your first oils from different families:

Citrus: bergamot, grapefruit, lemon, lime, mandarin, orange

Floral: geranium, chamomile (Roman), rose otto (or rose phytol), lavender

Herbaceous: chamomile (Roman), lavender, peppermint, rosemary, tea tree

Camphoraceous*: eucalyptus, cajeput, rosemary, peppermint, tea tree

Spicy: coriander, black pepper, ginger, cardamom

Resinous: frankincense, elemi, myrrh, galbanum

Woody: cedarwood (Virginian), sandalwood, pine, juniper berry, cypress

Earthy: patchouli, vetiver

*Homeopaths disagree about the effect of aromatherapy on homeopathy. Some believe there is no interaction, others believe that oils from this family can neutralize homeopathic medicines, and others believe that all aromatherapy oils can neutralize homeopathic medicines. If you are using aromatherapy at the same time as homeopathy, discuss this with your homeopath.

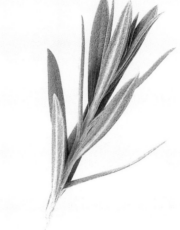

Lavender

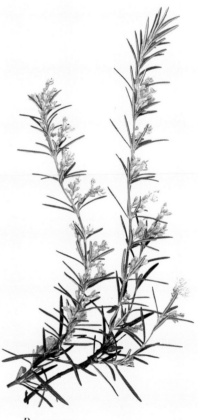

Rosemary

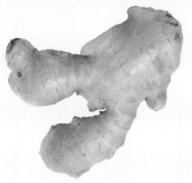

Ginger

Caring for your oils

Most essential oils, including bergamot, will keep for several years. The other citrus oils may deteriorate within nine months. Once oils have been blended with a base oil (see Massage, pages 122–3) they keep for about two months if stored correctly in dark colored glass bottles, at a cool temperature, in a dark place.

What are essential oils?

Essential oils are the aromatic liquids found in plants. They are sometimes known as essences or volatile oils and, as the latter name suggests, they evaporate very quickly if left in the open air. Essential oils are contained in different parts of the plants, including the flower petals (rose), leaves (eucalyptus), seeds (caraway), and bulbs (garlic). The price reflects the amount of oil that is available for extraction in any particular plant, and this varies greatly.

A number of methods are used to extract the oil from the plant, and the quality of the oil depends to some extent on the method used. One of the oldest methods is distillation in which the plant material is exposed to steam. The steam is then condensed to hot water and the captured essential oil is distilled from the water. A number of other solvents, including carbon dioxide under pressure, can also be used. Certain oils are extracted by applying pressure – for example, oils from citrus fruits are obtained simply by squeezing the peel.

Buy your oils from a reputable company because adulteration is common, and the label should state that the oil is 100 percent essential oil. The word *aromatherapy* is often applied to products that have an aroma but contain very little, if any, essential oil. Although prediluted oils seem to be less expensive, they can work out to be more costly than undiluted oil because they are not strong enough to be used by the drop to perfume a bath, for example. A whole bottle is likely to provide insufficient essence for more than one massage.

The benefits of aromatherapy

At a basic level, you can use aromatherapy to help you relax or to provide stimulation and invigoration. The symptoms of short-term acute illnesses, such as coughs and colds, will also often respond well to simple aromatherapy. However, for more chronic problems the help of a professional aromatherapist is recommended.

Conditions that can be treated with the help of a professional aromatherapist include:

- Depression and anxiety.

- Painful muscles and joints.

- Digestive disorders.

Aromatherapy oils can be used in your bath to enhance a good night's sleep.

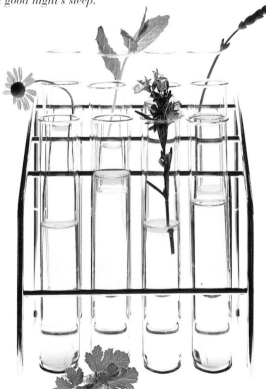

- Respiratory conditions including asthma.

- Menopause and vaginal yeast infections.

- Skin conditions, including cold sores and athlete's foot.

- Circulatory problems.

- Headaches.

(This list is not intended to be comprehensive. It is best to make a preliminary inquiry about your own condition, or ask your doctor's advice.)

Using aromatherapy oils

Aromatherapy can be applied in a number of ways:

- *Aromatic baths:* for pleasure, to enhance restful sleep, for skin problems or painful muscles, for relaxation, or for stimulation. Sprinkle up to eight drops of essential oil onto the surface of the bathwater and agitate the water to disperse the oil. If you have sensitive skin, use only one or two drops. If you have dry skin, you may wish to dissolve the essential oil into a base oil, such as sweet almond, but this will leave the tub greasy. For relaxation, have a warm bath, at about body temperature, and use chamomile or lavender. For stimulation, have a cooler bath and add pine, rosemary, or eucalyptus. You can also use aromatherapy oils with hydrotherapy (see page 140). If you prefer to have a shower, put two or three drops of oil onto a facecloth or sponge and rub it over your body as you shower.

- *Sauna:* clear your airways by inhaling the vapors from the oil. Mix just two drops of essential oil into about 2⅓ cups (600ml) of water and pour onto a heat source. Do not be tempted to use more or the aroma will be overwhelming. Appropriate oils include eucalyptus, lemon, peppermint, or pine. It is best to avoid sweet-smelling oils, such as rose and geranium. (Caution: saunas are not suitable if you have heart or lung disorders.)

- *Inhalations:* to clear the nasal passages when you have a cold, place 5–10 drops of an oil onto your handkerchief or pillow, or put a few drops onto a dampened absorbent cotton ball and place this on a radiator. This will also freshen a stuffy room. To make a steam inhalation, place a couple of drops into about 2 cups (500ml) of hot, but not boiling, water and inhale the steam.

- *Massage oils:* essential oils need to be diluted in a base oil before they can be used in a massage. Many oils are suitable for a base, and common examples are olive, almond, safflower, or sunflower. These should be labeled either "unrefined" or "cold pressed." Remember to test them if you have sensitive

Safety first: testing your skin

Even if you do not have sensitive skin, it is a good idea to do a skin test before using any oil that you have not used before. If your skin is sensitive such a test is essential. Mix one drop of the essential oil that you wish to test in a teaspoonful of a base oil that you know to be safe. Rub some onto an area of the skin that is particularly sensitive, such as behind the ear, the front of the wrist, or the inside of the elbow. Do not cover or wash the area for 24 hours and then check to see if the skin is red or feels itchy. If not, the oil is safe for you to use.

Light and color therapies

Light and color therapies are based on the belief that light and color can influence the sensory system of the body since they can be seen through the eyes. Many people say they feel much better on a bright day than on a dull one, and this is thought to be to result of the influence of light on the body's energy. In winter, especially in colder countries, the lack of natural light is thought to lead to depression, fatigue, and overeating. People most deeply affected can develop seasonal affective disorder (SAD), which may respond to light therapy. Normal daylight provides a full spectrum of color, plus ultraviolet and infrared colors that cannot be seen by the human eye. Color therapists believe light and color change the internal balance of the body, and work with colors to restore disturbed balance.

skin (see left). Base oils generally keep for about nine months in a refrigerator or other cool place. Massage oils are usually diluted at a rate between 0.5 and 2 percent, using the weakest mixture for sensitive skin. For 0.5 percent you will need one drop of essential oil in 2 teaspoons (10ml) of base oil, and for 2 percent you will need 2 drops of essential oil in 1 teaspoon (5ml) of base oil. For a full body massage you will need about 6 teaspoons (30ml) of oil, or a little more for hairy or dry skin. (For massage techniques, see page 121.)

Cautions
- Keep essential oils out of the reach of children.

- Do not apply undiluted essential oils to the skin (apart from lavender oil for minor burns and cuts).

- Keep essential oils away from your eyes.

- Never take essential oils orally, unless a doctor or qualified aromatherapist prescribes them.

- Beware of using essential oils in a sauna or diffuser. Severe allergic reactions of the skin and respiratory system can occur with large exposure to oils. Read the instructions that come with the diffuser.

- Keep oils away from varnished surfaces.

- Citrus oils can make the skin more sensitive to sunlight: avoid these shortly before exposing your skin to sunlight or a tanning bed; if you have had a melanoma or other skin cancer; or if you have age spots, large moles, warts, or many freckles.

- Avoid using the same oil for longer than three months without taking a break of about two months because it is possible for your skin to become sensitive to the oil. If you have sensitive skin always test your skin before using any oil that you have not used before.

- If you have epilepsy, avoid the essential oils of rosemary, fennel, and sage.

- Extra precautions are necessary if you wish to try aromatherapy with children or pregnant women.

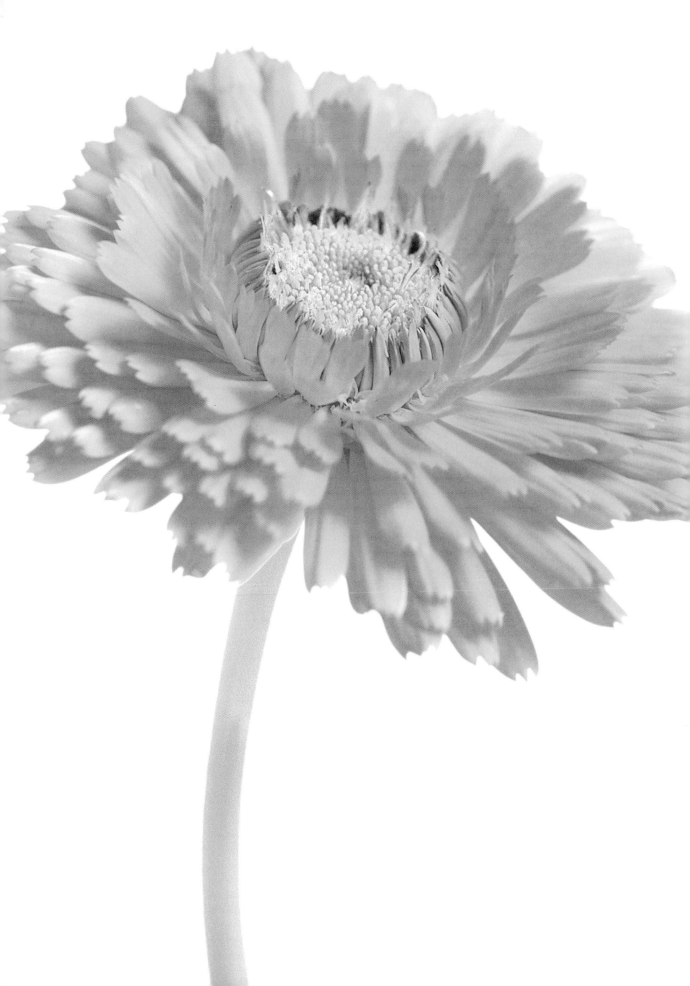

Chapter Seven

ENERGY

Many alternative practitioners believe that we have a vital inner energy within the body, and that illness occurs when this energy is blocked or becomes unbalanced in some way. Although this energy cannot be scientifically defined or understood as yet, reestablishing an inner balance of energy is a recurring theme in many of the complementary medical systems described in this book.

"Live all you can; it's a mistake not to."

Henry James (1843–1916)

AYURVEDIC
MEDICINE

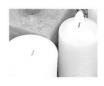

Ayurveda means "the knowledge of life." It is one of the oldest and most complete medical systems, and Indian scholars date its origins to around 6,000 BC. Ayurvedic physicians (at this point there is no government licensing of Ayurvedic practitioners in North America) believe that health reflects the harmonious operation of the body, mind, and soul, and that disease is caused when an imbalance occurs. Ayurvedic medicine is part of a complex philosophy, which most conventionally trained health-care practitioners today would not consider to be an integral part of healing.

In Ayurveda the human being is regarded as a microcosm of the universe. The five elements of the universe correspond to the five senses of the body and five modes of action (see box, right). The life force, known as *prana*, is controlled by three basic forces, or *doshas*, which exist in all things and function in human beings as follows: *pit*, or bodily fire, controls the biochemical functions of the body; *kaph*, or biological water, controls the fluid metabolism of the body and certain psychological functions; *vat*, or bodily air, controls movement and the nervous system. Diseases occur when these forces are not in balance within the individual.

Polarity therapy

Polarity therapy, developed by Randolf Stone (a chiropractor, osteopath, and naturopath) in the 1950s, is based on the Ayurvedic principle that health and happiness depend on the free flow of energy between the five chakras, the energy centers of the body. Therapy includes the use of touch, the development of psychological awareness, cleansing diets, and gentle exercises.

Ayurvedic elements, senses, and actions

Element	Sense	Organ	Action	Vehicle of action
Space or ether	Hearing	Ear	Speech	Mouth
Air	Touch	Skin	Holding, giving, receiving	Hand
Fire	Vision	Eye	Walking	Feet
Water	Taste	Tongue	Procreation	Genitals
Earth	Smell	Nose	Excretion	Anus

Ayurvedic practice

Various therapeutic methods are used in Ayurvedic medicine, and specialties, such as surgery, have developed in much the same way as in modern conventional medicine. Treatment is chosen to match both the constitution of the patient and the particular illness that has occurred.

There is great emphasis on diet, both for its direct effect on the patient and also for its influence on the action of any medicine that might be prescribed. It is believed that an inappropriate diet can cause the accumulation of toxic substances. These are called *ama* and are thought to cause disease by disturbing the natural balance of the body. As a result, dietary changes, including the use of fasting, are usually recommended at the start of treatment.

Yoga (see page 126), meditation (see page 150), chanting, attention to posture, sleep, and other aspects of lifestyle are also usually included in an initial prescription. Herbal medicines may be recommended, and again these are chosen specifically for the individual. They may be prescribed to be taken at particular times during the day, a concept that has only recently begun to be developed in modern conventional treatment.

Stronger treatments may be required if the disease fails to respond to the initial therapy. These include purification by inducing diarrhea or vomiting, and surgery. These treatments are recognized to be potentially weakening and so, when the disease has been eliminated, rejuvenation therapy is prescribed to restore full balance and strength.

Medication

The Ayurvedic pharmacy is highly developed and complex. There are more than 8,000 preparations, most of which are derived from plants and minerals. Some of the substances used have been subjected to modern research and found to have pharmacological properties relevant for the disease for which they are prescribed. For example, cumin, which is given for rheumatic conditions, contains curcurmin, which has anti-inflammatory properties.

It is also possible that some Ayurvedic medicines may have useful properties that, so far, the pharmaceutical industry has been unable to recreate. These include substances that may protect the body from the side effects of drugs that suppress the immune system, often used after transplant surgery, or to protect the liver from overdoses of acetaminophen.

TRADITIONAL **CHINESE** MEDICINE

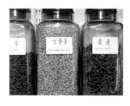

Traditional Chinese medicine, which is a complete medical system, has been practiced for centuries and contains a number of similarities to Ayurvedic medicine, partly due to the influence of Buddhism. Chinese medical practice includes acupuncture and acupressure (see page 162), moxibustion (see page 165), the use of herbs, cupping (see box, right), and attention to lifestyle and diet.

In traditional Chinese medicine there is a belief that health is maintained when there is a balance between the mind, the body, and the outside world. The causes of illness can therefore come from unresolved emotional problems, from a stressful lifestyle, from smoking or eating too much, or from external factors, such as climatic conditions.

Qi: the vital energy

The idea that blood circulates through the body is familiar to Western society, and the Chinese believe that the vital energy or Qi (pronounced chee) circulates in a similar fashion along energy pathways known as meridians. Most of these are connected to the major organs of the body, and their existence has been confirmed by electrical measurement. In addition, the organs of the body are related to the five elements: wind, water, earth, fire, and metal, and these too have to be in balance for health.

The universal forces of yin and yang are thought to regulate Qi. These are interdependent forces that represent opposite qualities, yet each contains a seed of the other.

Yang qualities	Yin qualities
Heat	Coldness
Strength	Weakness
Light	Darkness
Expansion	Contraction
Above	Below
Back	Front

It is believed that ill, coldness, pallor, and fatigue indicate the yin state, while a fever, causing heat and a flushed appearance, indicates the yang state. The basis of treatment is to restore the balance between yin and yang.

Chinese herbalism

Chinese herbalism has probably been practiced for 4,000 years. Prior to the writing of the first textbook in the sixteenth century many of the recipes were handed on from parent to child. The raw ingredients of Chinese "herbs" consist of dried materials derived from plants, but may also include animal products and minerals. They are classified according to their properties, such as being warming or cooling.

Chinese medicine

Cupping

Cupping is thought to remove any wind, cold, or damp that may be trapped in the body, and is commonly used to relieve swollen and painful joints, and to treat the early phases of colds or the flu. The cups are made from glass, bamboo, metal, or ceramics. A lighted taper or match is placed briefly inside the cup to create a vacuum before placing it on the skin. The vacuum increases the flow of blood to the skin in the area under the cup. More than one cup at a time may be used, and they are usually left in place for up to 15 minutes, before being removed by pressing the adjacent skin to break the vacuum.

Chinese herbs

Traditional combinations of herbs are cooked and made into medicinal soups, which are often bitter. Historically, the recipes were changed according to the patient's progress. More recently, however, fixed combinations have been produced in factories in forms more acceptable to the Western palate. Where these fixed combinations are used, regrettably some of the flexibility of prescribing for the individual has been lost. Chinese herbs are useful for the treatment of a wide range of ailments, including asthma, skin diseases, migraines, and digestive disturbances.

Chinese herbs have become very popular in the West, but some problems have arisen where medicines have sometimes lacked adequate quality control. If you want to use Chinese herbs you should ensure that they come from a reputable source. Herbs from Taiwan, the US and Britain have fewer quality-control problems.

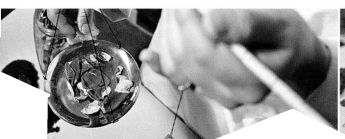
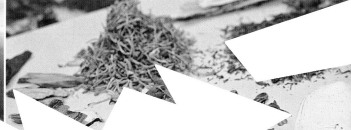

ACUPUNCTURE AND ACUPRESSURE

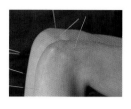

Acupuncture originated in China and is an integral part of traditional Chinese medicine (see page 160). Acupuncture usually involves the insertion of very thin needles into the skin to adjust the flow of energy in the body. The needles are inserted at carefully selected "points" in the meridians, or energy channels. These points have been likened to whirlpools of energy that develop where the energy flow along the meridian is disrupted. Some of the points are tender when pressed, but acupuncturists find others by using methods of measurement that have been developed over many centuries. It is believed that the insertion of the needles and their gentle manipulation disperses stagnant energy and restores the normal energy balance.

In China, acupuncture is used to maintain health rather than treat illness, but in the West few people consult an acupuncturist until something has gone wrong, and usually not until other treatment has failed. Despite this delay, acupuncture can often heal or alleviate the problem.

Scientific acupuncture

Some acupuncturists believe that acupuncture can be explained in terms of modern scientific knowledge, ignoring the traditional belief in the meridians. They accept that it has long been noticed in the West that the gentle massage of small areas of tenderness on the skin can relieve pain in distant parts of the body. These areas have been likened to acupuncture points, and practitioners of "scientific acupuncture" believe that the Chinese have developed the recognition of these points far more extensively than in the West. Scientific acupuncturists use Chinese acupuncture points without accepting the underlying philosophy of Chinese medicine (briefly described on pages 160–161).

The acupuncture needles

Acupuncture needles are made of stainless steel, silver, or gold, and many practitioners now use disposable needles. If needles already used on you are to be reused, however, they should be

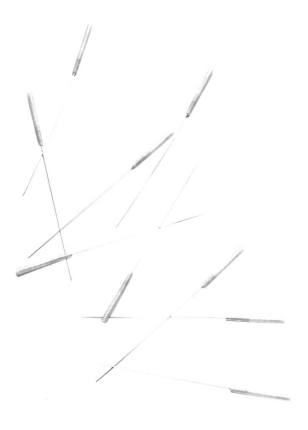

Acupuncture needles are solid and much finer than the hollow needles used for injections.

minutes. The size of the needles varies according to the site where they are used. Longer, larger needles are inserted more deeply into fleshy areas, such as the buttocks. Finer, shorter needles are used for areas where the flesh is thin, such as the forehead. The acupuncture points that are chosen may remain the same at each treatment, but they may need to be changed when the patient's health alters or improves.

The acupuncture consultation

The initial diagnosis can take up to an hour and you will be asked:

■ To provide information about your current problem(s), your medical history, and that of your family. The acupuncturist will also want to know more about how your body is functioning generally, such as how you are sleeping, whether you have any other symptoms or health problems – either physical or psychological – and how you react to heat or cold. The acupuncturist will also assess your psychological health.

sterilized first. Make sure that the practitioner never uses needles that were used on another patient first.

Acupuncture needles come in various sizes, but they are all solid and much finer than the hollow needles used for injections. They have rounded tips, which divide the flesh, rather than piercing it. When inserted they rarely cause bleeding. In general, acupuncture sessions last 20 to 45

■ To undergo a physical examination. This may be similar to an examination by your doctor, but acupuncturists often examine your tongue in greater detail and use the Chinese method of assessing the pulse. This is more complex than a conventional Western examination, because it includes feeling the wrist pulse in 12 different positions and noting up to 28 different aspects of the pulse.

Tai chi

Tai chi consists of a sequence of gentle flowing movements that are precisely performed, and coordinated with breathing. Conventional scientific studies have revealed that tai chi can have benefits that are similar to aerobic exercise, but with less physical stress and strain. It can benefit high blood pressure, insomnia, anxiety, muscle tension, and various other causes of chronic ill health.

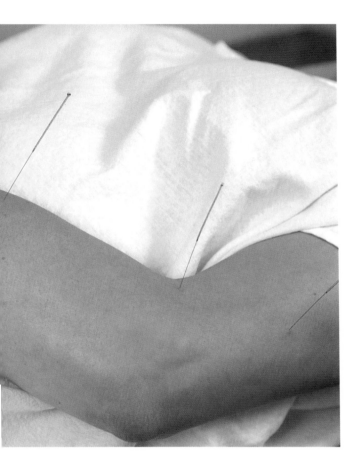

Acupuncture needles can be left in place for up to 20 minutes.

Assessing the results

Some patients feel a change immediately after treatment but others only become aware of results after a number of sessions. It is often difficult to remember exactly how you felt at the start of treatment; your therapist may jog your memory by reminding you of how you described your initial symptoms. Your acupuncturist will assess your progress by observing your appearance and manner as well as by reexamining your pulse.

The number of sessions that are needed varies from person to person. Acute symptoms usually clear up within four treatments, but chronic conditions generally take longer.

Conditions where acupuncture may be helpful:

- Respiratory problems.

- Arthritis and rheumatism.

- Circulatory problems.

- Digestive disturbances.

- Ear, nose, and throat problems.

- Menopausal symptoms.

- Mental and emotional problems.

- Urinary problems.

(This list is not intended to be comprehensive. It is best to make a preliminary inquiry about your own condition, or ask your doctor's advice.)

The acupuncturist will then decide whether acupuncture is an appropriate treatment. Acupuncturists who are fully trained in traditional Chinese medicine may also prescribe herbal treatment. In addition to the use of acupuncture needles, your therapist may suggest cupping (see page 161) or moxibustion (see opposite).

Chi kung

Chi kung (pronounced chee goong) is an ancient Eastern exercise that is believed to aid the free flow of energy through the body by means of movement and balance. This allows healing to occur and good health to be maintained. The chi kung practitioner aims to avoid stress on the joints and muscles and encourages an inner awareness of the movement of energy within the body. It can help overcome stress, sexual problems, and conditions associated with aging.

Cautions

Acupuncture should never be performed on a person with a high fever, or who is under the influence of either alcohol or an illicit drug. Acupuncture should be done with caution on patients taking blood-thinning medication. It is a safe treatment when performed by a fully qualified practitioner who takes special care when treating elderly or frail people. If you are concerned about the use of unsterile needles, discuss this with your acupuncturist, who will be able to explain the procedure he or she follows.

Auricular therapy

Acupuncture points on the ear are used for auricular therapy, either alone or in conjunction with the acupuncture points elsewhere on the body. It is most often used for the treatment of addiction or the relief of pain. The acupuncture points on the ear have to be very carefully located. There are more than 300 auricular points and they are very close together. Small needles are used and they are sometimes kept in place for a few days with surgical adhesive tape.

A weak electrical current is sometimes used to stimulate the acupuncture points on the ear, but other points elsewhere on the body are also sometimes stimulated in this way. Since the 1950s, techniques of electroacupuncture have been used in China to provide anesthesia for surgery. This form of anesthesia is of particular benefit for surgery of the upper part of the body. It is also useful for old or frail patients since it is less risky than conventional anesthesia, and the recovery time is usually quicker.

Moxibustion

Moxibustion is a technique that is used to supply warmth. The affected part of the body may be described as feeling cold, or the pain may have been relieved by the application of heat, such as in a warm bath or with a hot water bottle. The herb moxa is also used to nourish Qi (vital energy, see page 160) and the blood, when the symptoms include general weakness and a lack of energy.

Moxibustion involves burning a small amount of the herb moxa (*Artemisia vulgaris*), also known as mugwort, in one of four ways:

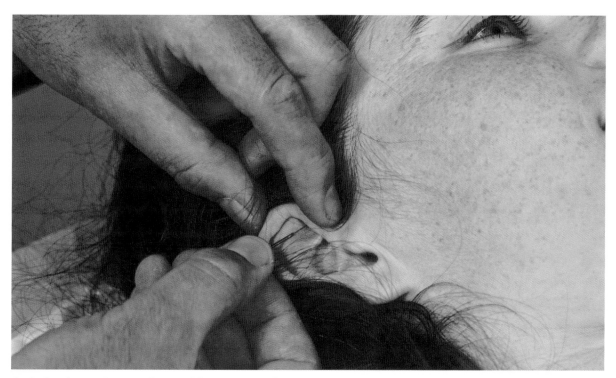

Auricular therapy is most often used for treatment of addiction or relief of pain.

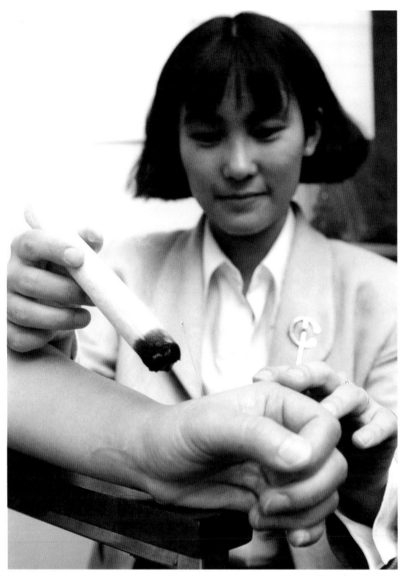

A moxa stick being used by a therapist to relieve pain.

■ To replenish energy, cones of moxa are allowed to smolder on specific points on the skin (called direct moxa), being removed by the therapist when heat is felt by the patient. This treatment can cause scarring and many experts recommend against it.

■ When the therapist wishes to apply heat to a larger area, moxa is burned in a box placed on the appropriate area of skin.

■ A moxa stick is lit before being held over the body to warm it. This method of moxibustion can also be done by the patient at home.

Using a moxa stick

The moxa stick looks somewhat like a cigar, and is best lit from a candle, which can take about half a minute. Ash will form as you are using it, and this should be tapped off into an ashtray. The lit stick is then held over the skin at a distance that provides you with comfortable warmth. You may choose to move the stick closer to the skin with a dabbing movement for extra warmth, but you should take care not to burn the skin. Once the area being treated feels warm you

■ The dried herb is attached to an acupuncture needle already inserted in the skin and then lit to supply deep heat.

Seitei

Seitei is an Eastern combination of acupressure, manipulation, and nutritional therapy. It is based on the theory that the body can be made stronger if its energy system is stimulated, and that the correct nutritional support enables the body to heal any structural problems more quickly.

can move to another area, or extinguish the stick by cutting off the end. You can use moxibustion once or twice a week, but take a couple of weeks off every month or so. The application of moxa should be relaxing and pleasurable: if it is not, you should not continue to use it.

Cautions

Moxibustion is generally safe. However, it should not be used:

- To treat inflamed tissues or during acute illness, especially if you have a fever.

- If you have a skin rash or if the skin is broken, cut, or grazed.

- If you have high blood pressure.

- If you find that the smoke given off by the burning herb is an irritant.

- Near sensitive skin, such as on the face.

Acupressure

Like acupuncture, acupressure uses the points on the energy meridians, but here they are stimulated by the application of gentle pressure either in a sustained manner, intermittently (by alternately pressing and releasing), or with small massage movements. Acupressure is related to massage (see page 120), reflexology (see page 172), and shiatsu (see page 176). Acupressure classes are offered by many HMOs.

Promote your health

The most important role for acupressure is the maintenance of health although, as with acupuncture, a professional therapist can use the technique for treatment. It is most effective when it is used frequently and for short periods and is therefore a therapy that is ideally suited for self-treatment. Your therapist may teach you how to continue the treatment he or she has started. Or, you may start to apply acupressure after learning the positions of the acupoints from a book or even a friend. Once you have gained confidence you will be able to use the acupoints for immediate first-aid treatment for acute conditions, as well as for maintaining your health.

Conditions that may be helped by acupressure include:

- Headaches.

- Back pain.

- Constipation.

- Asthma.

- Fatigue.

(This list is not intended to be comprehensive. It is best to make a preliminary inquiry about your own condition, or ask your doctor's advice.)

Cautions

Acupressure can alter symptoms and may mask the early symptoms of serious conditions, such as cancer. You should, therefore, seek advice from your doctor before consulting a therapist for any condition other than an acute problem, such as a cold or a cough, so that an accurate diagnosis can be made. Always start treatment very gently, especially if you are feeling weak or fatigued. Acupressure should never be used when you are under the influence of alcohol or nonmedicinal drugs. Acupressure must not be practiced on broken or inflamed skin, or over scars, bruises, or veins that are enlarged or painful.

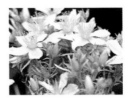

HOMEOPATHY

Modern homeopathy, which was founded by Samuel Hahnemann (1755–1843), is based on two principles. The first is that "like cures like." In other words, medicine given to an ill person can cure the same symptoms that it causes when given to a healthy person. The second principle is that the minimum necessary dose should be given, to avoid causing harm. The first principle was not new; Hippocrates taught it more than 4,000 years earlier. Hahnemann proved it on himself, however, when he took low doses of quinine and developed the symptoms of malaria. In fact, quinine is used even today to treat malaria.

Hahnemann was disillusioned by the medical practice of his day, which included the administration of very toxic substances, such as mercury. He built on his experience of taking quinine by giving small doses of medicinal substances to healthy people and carefully noting the symptoms that each substance produced. He then used the medicine to treat people who suffered from the same symptoms that the medical substance had produced in a healthy person.

Although many of his patients recovered, they initially responded to their medicine with increased symptoms. To avoid this Hahnemann reduced the dose that he prescribed, but the medicine then became ineffective.

Hahnemann was sure that he could find a way around this problem and started to reduce the dose in a different way. He diluted one drop of medicine in 10 drops of water and shook it vigorously before taking one drop of that mixture and diluting it in another 10 drops of water, and repeating the process several more times. To his surprise, the medicine appeared to become more powerful, and he called this process "potentization." Homeopathic medicines are prepared in a similar way today, and the degree of dilution is usually called the "potency."

The homeopathic consultation

The first consultation with a homeopath will often take around an hour because homeopaths believe that family history and inherited characteristics should be considered, along with the physical, mental, and emotional characteristics that have been acquired by your experience of life. These can include what you like or dislike eating, whether you are thirsty, what sort of weather you prefer, your fears, whether you are tidy, a spendthrift, or a saver.

The homeopath will want to know about your symptoms in ways that differ from a consultation with a conventional doctor. It is important to discover what makes the symptoms better or worse, when they occur, whether there were any great upheavals in your life when they started, and how your illness is affecting you emotionally. In addition your homeopath may ask questions about the times when you are well. Taken together, these characteristics are considered to indicate the "constitutional" type of the patient.

Your constitutional type can change during your life, and even to the most experienced homeopath it is not always clear. Some people show characteristics of more than one constitutional type. Other people may truly need more than one prescription to become healthy again, although many homeopaths prefer to give just one prescription when possible.

What can homeopathy treat?

Homeopathy can be used to treat almost any complaint that can be treated with conventional medicine, as opposed to one requiring surgery. Chronic conditions, such as eczema, psoriasis, headaches, allergies, digestive disorders, such as irritable bowel syndrome and chronic fatigue syndrome, and psychological disorders, such as anxiety or depression, are best treated with

constitutional prescriptions. However, many people become very good at treating their own acute illnesses, such as coughs, colds, stomach upsets, and minor injuries (see the homeopathic first-aid box, page 171).

What do homeopathic medicines look like?

Homeopathic medicines are made up in liquid form, usually with alcohol as a preservative. This is dropped onto tablets, granules, or powders that are usually made from lactose. If you are lactose intolerant you can ask the pharmacist to use a different sugar. It is also possible to have the medicine prepared in liquid form in alcohol or water, but the latter has a very short shelf life. In the United States, homeopathic products must meet over-the-counter "good manufacturing practices for drugs." So quality control is far superior to that of dietary supplements, including herbal products. But unlike OTC drug manufacturers,

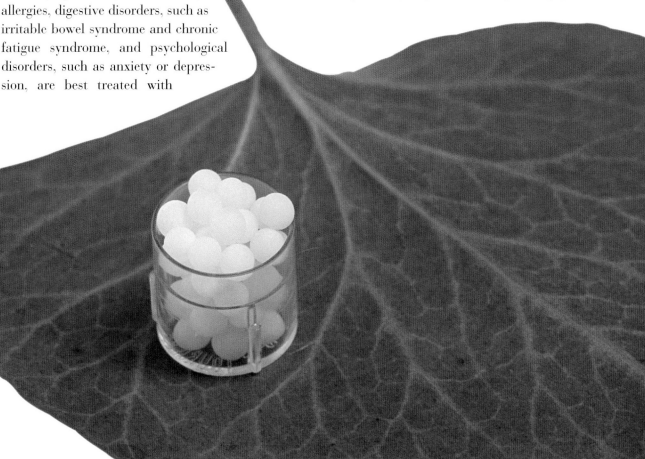

Homeopathic treatments can be used to treat many medical problems, except those that require surgery.

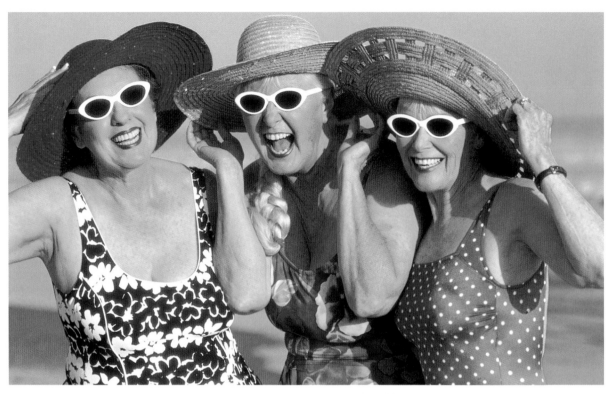

Homeopathy can restore health and a sense of well-being without causing side effects.

homeopathic products are not required to show that their products are effective.

Cautions and side effects
Homeopathic medicines are very safe for people of all ages but if, as sometimes occurs, your symptoms become worse, you should stop taking the medicine. This aggravation will generally reduce within a few days, and often then disappear. Sometimes you will develop new symptoms, which you should keep track of because they can help your homeopath choose your next prescription.

The legislation governing who can practice homeopathy varies from one country to another, and some homeopaths are also conventionally trained doctors. If you consult a homeopath who is not a doctor, it is wise for your own doctor to make the diagnosis since other treatment may be more appropriate.

Self-help with homeopathy
Homeopathy can be used to treat common everyday ailments very safely. Many people buy homeopathic medicines to treat simple conditions as they arise, and gradually build up a stock of different medicines. To remain effective, the medicines must be stored in closed containers. These should be kept in the dark, and away from perfumes and other aromatic substances, especially mothballs.

Schuessler mineral salts

Schuessler mineral salts (also known as biochemic salts) consist of 12 of the minerals that occur naturally in the tissues of the body. They are prepared in the same way as homeopathic medicines, but only to a low potency (see page 168), and they are used in a similar way.

Suggestions for your homeopathic first-aid box

Argentum nitricum Anxiety or fear when anticipating a big event

Arnica Shock after injury to yourself or someone else; jet lag, bruising, sprained joints, strained or torn muscles

Arsenicum album Fear or panic when you are alone; diarrhea and vomiting occurring together

Bryonia Swollen joints that are painful when you move; painful dry cough

Calendula ointment Heals and prevents infetion in cuts and grazes

Gelsemium The flu with chills, when the head and body feel heavy; anxiety and confusion before an important event

Glonoine Heat exhaustion, bursting headaches, or menopausal hot flashes

Hypericum Pain from crushed nerves, such as a crushed fingertip

Ignatia Shock or grief from bad news

Ledum Puncture wounds such as insect bites, or after an injection

Natrum mur The effects of grief or bereavement; a cold or hayfever with sneezing and a clear nasal discharge

Nux vomica The effects of eating or drinking too much; insomnia from mental strain

Pulsatilla Sinusitis with yellow bland nasal discharge; the effects of a sudden soaking

Rhus tox Arthritis that is worse in cold, damp weather, but better after a very hot bath; cold sores, shingles (in addition to medical advice)

Urtica ointment Minor burns and scalds, skin allergies, and insect bites and stings

The potency most readily available over the counter is usually labeled 6 or 6c, and it is safest to start with this. In acute conditions take a dose every 30 minutes for up to six doses, but decrease the frequency as the symptoms improve. You may then need to take a dose three times a day for a few days, but you should stop when your symptoms relent. If there has been no improvement after six doses you will need to change the medicine. In chronic conditions, such as arthritis, take two or three doses a day when symptoms are present and none when they are absent.

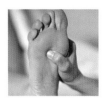

REFLEXOLOGY

Reflexology is a specific form of massage that is usually applied to the feet, but it can also be used on the hands. It has probably been in use for at least 5,000 years, and is depicted on the frieze of the 4,000-year-old tomb of an Egyptian doctor. The Inca and Native Americans used various forms of foot massage. In fact, it may have been observation of the latter that inspired the American physician, Dr. William Fitzgerald, whose work laid the foundations of modern reflexology.

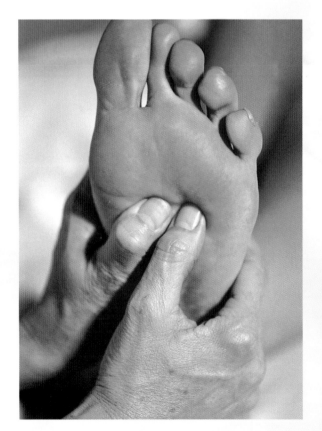

Fitzgerald believed that the body can be divided into 10 energy zones, five on each side. These zones start at the big toe (zone 1) and run up through the body to the head. He believed that stimulation of one zone on the foot or the hand affects other parts of the body that belong to the same zone. The work was continued by one of Fitzgerald's assistants, Eunice Ingham. She developed a complete body chart illustrating the body zones on the feet. These zones are known as reflex points.

How does reflexology work?

In the philosophy of many therapeutic systems it is believed that the life force or energy (Qi, see page 160, or *prana*, see page 158) flows in the body, and that illness occurs when the movement of this energy is obstructed. Reflexologists believe that blockage is caused by crystalline calcium

Reflexology is a popular therapy that can help stress disorders, headaches, and digestive problems.

deposits forming on the end of nerves as a result of congestion, inflammation, or other disorder in the nerve pathways. The resulting blockage is removed when pressure is applied to the reflex points mapped out on the feet and hands.

Little scientific research has been done to prove the theories of reflexology. It is a popular non-invasive therapy that appears to be reasonably safe in the hands of nontherapists, who can give valuable health support. For treatment, however, it is best to consult a professional therapist.

Conditions that can be treated by a professional reflexologist include:

- Digestive problems.

- Stress and stress-related disorders, including fatigue and palpitations.

- Various aches and pains, including back pain and repetitive strain injury.

- Certain skin conditions.

- Migraines and other headaches.

- Ear problems, including tinnitus.

- Sinus problems and rhinitis.

- Various chest problems, including asthma.

- Chronic conditions affecting the elderly, such as dementia.

(This list is not intended to be comprehensive. It is best to make a preliminary inquiry about your own condition, or ask your doctor's advice.)

Cautions

Reflexology should not be used when thrombosis is present. Some therapists advise against the use of reflexology on people with arthritis, osteoporosis, or disorders of the heart or thyroid gland.

The consultation

The therapist takes a history of your past and present health problems, usually including your lifestyle. You will be asked to sit or lie in a comfortable position in a peaceful atmosphere in order to undergo treatment; the therapy is most effective when you are relaxed.

Your therapist will check for corns, calluses, and other areas that might be painful when pressure is applied. Treatment consists of the firm application of pressure to the reflex points on the feet. Various movements are used, such as rubbing and rotating with the pads of the thumbs and fingers over small areas at any one time. Eastern practitioners may use a sharpened stick

Vacuflex reflexology system

The **Vacuflex reflexology system** was devised during the 1970s by a Danish reflexologist, Inge Dougans, who believed that reflexology is more closely related to the Eastern meridians (see page 162) than to the zones proposed by Dr. William Fitzgerald. There are two stages to vacuflex reflexology. In the first stage special boots are fitted to the feet. When the air inside the boots is pumped out, the feet are squeezed, so that all the reflex points are stimulated at the same time. The vacuum is maintained for about five minutes. The boots are then removed and the therapist has about half a minute to examine the feet and note any yellow or red color changes on them. These are believed to indicate which parts of the body are in need of treatment. The therapist then places silicon pads along the appropriate meridian lines of all the limbs, using a number of different sizes of pad. These are briefly held in place by suction, which is thought to provide sufficient stimulation for healing to occur.

and other practitioners apply a vacuum (see box, page 173). The therapist usually maintains constant touch, while working methodically over the areas to be treated. Because it is impossible to apply pressure accurately if the skin is slippery, oils or creams are not used in reflexology. Sometimes a little powder is used.

A full reflexology session will take more than an hour. Initially the feet will be relaxed before being given a full workout. The hands are then treated. You are likely to feel some effects from your treatment as it is proceeding. Any pain or discomfort that results from "congestion" of the energy force is usually brief, and followed by a feeling of release. Most people feel light and relaxed immediately after a treatment, as well as having more energy. However, this may be followed by symptoms, known as cleansing reactions, such as a headache, a runny nose, frequent urination, or a mild skin rash.

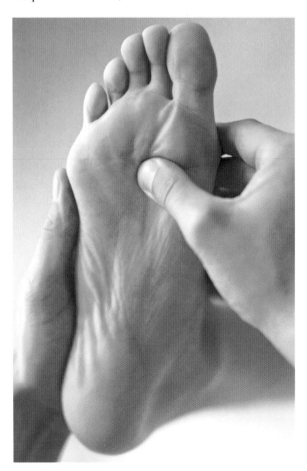

Reflexologists work to unblock crystalline calcium deposits that they believe form on the ends of nerves.

Relaxing your partner's feet

■ Your partner should be warm and comfortable with his or her feet supported at the level of your chest. If necessary, warm your hands.

■ "Greet the feet" by curving your hands over the top of them and holding them steadily for a minute or two.

■ Place your left thumb behind the toes of your partner's right foot to support the foot, leaving your fingers curled over the top of the foot. Using the thumb of your right hand massage the diaphragm line. This crosses the instep just below the ball of the foot and the solar plexus point (see below left). Make small circular movements, and each time you move the position of your thumb, rock the toes over your left thumb. Repeat on the left side.

■ Return to the right foot and massage each toe in turn between your thumbs and index fingers. Then gently move the toes up and down. Repeat on the left.

■ Cup the heel of the right foot in one hand, and, grasping the toes with the other hand, loosen the ankle joints by moving the foot up and down and then in a circular manner. Repeat on the left side.

■ Hold the sides of the left foot with your thumbs about 2 inches (5cm) apart. Gently stretch the top of the foot rather like breaking open a bread roll. Repeat on the right side.

■ Place one hand on the outside of each foot and press the solar plexus points firmly with your thumbs, using small rotational movements. (See where the thumb is positioned in the picture, left.)

■ Hold both feet again as in step 1 for a few minutes, allowing your partner to relax.

A full session will take more than an hour. Any discomfort will usually be followed by a feeling of release (right).

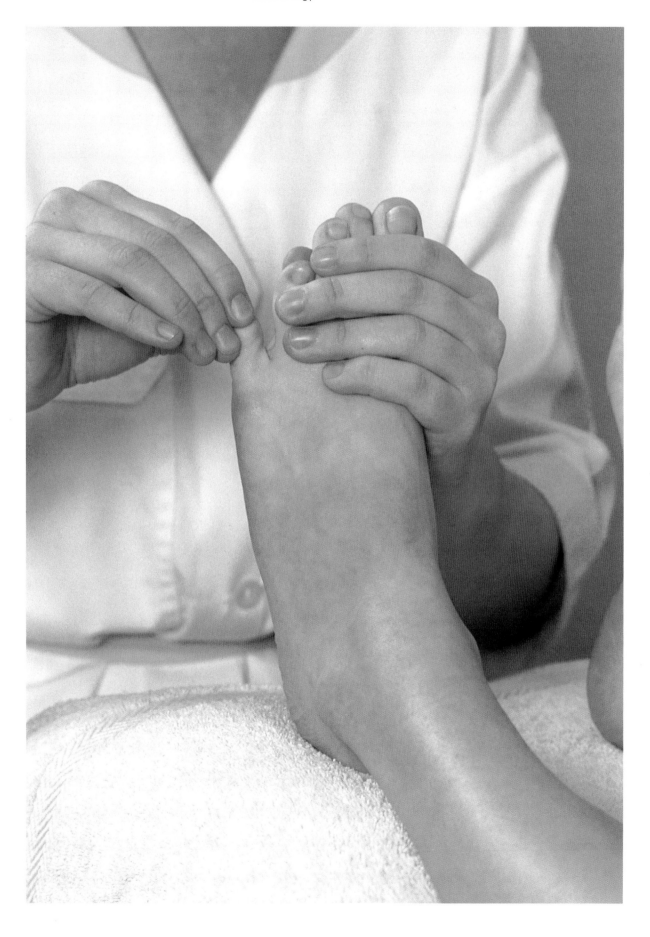

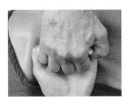

SHIATSU

The word *shiatsu* means finger pressure in Japanese, and the therapy of the same name has been called Japanese physical therapy. It is an ancient Eastern therapy in which sustained and stationary pressure is applied to the same points as those used in acupuncture and acupressure. In addition, the muscles are stretched to relieve muscular tension and various gentle manipulative techniques may also be included.

Shiatsu treatment

You will usually receive shiatsu lying on a mat on the floor or in the sitting position, and the pressure is applied through the clothing, so there is no need to undress. However, it is advisable to wear loose clothing to allow free movement as required.

The therapist makes a diagnosis of the areas of weakness by taking a history, examining the pulse, and palpating the abdomen. The treatment lasts between 60 and 90 minutes, and produces a feeling of deep relaxation and well-being.

You may experience healing reactions, such as flulike symptoms or a headache after the first treatment, but these usually last only a day or so, and become less and less marked as the course of treatment progresses.

You can receive shiatsu techniques from a friend to maintain health and reduce stress, but it is best to consult a practitioner if you require treatment for an ailment.

A course of shiatsu therapy usually involves four to eight sessions on a weekly basis, but many clients continue to have a maintenance treatment every month or so.

Conditions that can be treated by a professional shiatsu therapist include:

■ Digestive disorders, including constipation and diarrhea.

■ Back and neck pain.

■ Migraine and toothache.

■ Stress, tension, and mild depression.

■ Insomnia and disturbed sleep patterns. (This list is not intended to be comprehensive. It is best to make a preliminary inquiry about your own condition, or ask your doctor's advice.)

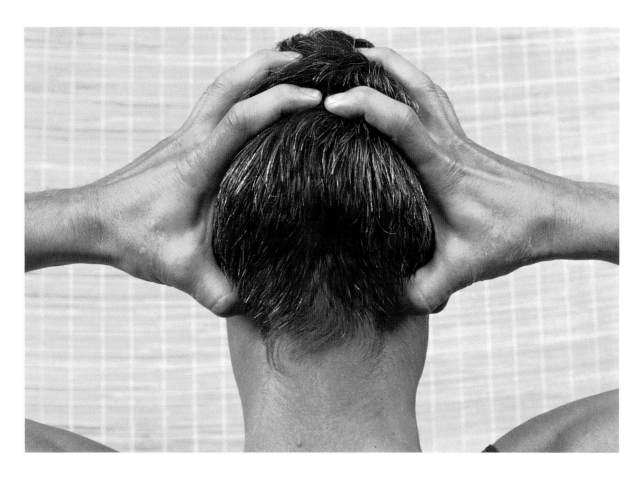

Shiatsu means finger pressure in Japanese.

Cautions

Shiatsu should not be given immediately after eating or when there is a high fever. Shiatsu is not applied to wounds, areas of inflammation, or scar tissue. It should be applied with caution to treat people with cancer, heart disease, or those who are elderly or frail.

Simple shiatsu for your partner

The following technique can be used to release tension in the neck. Sit your partner on the floor, on a rug or a cushion, and kneel behind.

- Place your hands on your partner's shoulders and pause briefly. Then start to squeeze and knead the trapezius muscle between your fingers and thumbs. This muscle connects the lower neck to the shoulders; you can feel it tighten if your partner shrugs his or her shoulders.

- Use a gentle chopping movement along the length of the muscle using the outer edge of your hand. You can increase the pressure, but make sure your partner does not experience undue discomfort.

- Kneel at the right side of your partner with your left knee supporting his or her back. Support your partner's forehead with your right hand, and using the thumb and fingers of your left hand knead the muscles at the back of the neck on both sides of the spine.

- Kneel behind your partner again and place your forearms on his or her shoulders. Apply gentle pressure by leaning forward. Ask your partner to take a deep breath, then as he or she breathes out, roll your arms outward toward the shoulders. Repeat several times.

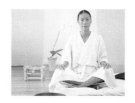

HEALING

Healing is the restoration of good health. Many alternative therapists believe that good health depends on the freedom with which energy flows through the body, and that therapy helps to free blockages and restore the imbalance that either causes or results from ill health.

Spiritual or psychic healing

Healing and healers are found in all the world's religions and also outside formal religious practice. Spiritual healing often occurs through the "laying on of hands," and during the past 30 years a number of nurses and other health-care professionals have been taught Therapeutic Touch, sometimes known as TT. Other healers provide a distant healing service and do not have a direct physical contact with their clients. People often experience the healing energy as a warm or cool feeling that promotes a sensation of well-being and relaxation.

Conditions that can be treated by a healer include:

■ Emotional, spiritual, and physical ailments.

■ Painful joints and muscles.

Cautions

Healing is a safe therapy, but you should avoid healers who demand substantial payment, or insist that you change your religious beliefs or abandon conventional medical treatment. The law in different countries can vary, especially regarding healing of children under 18. Healing should be obtained in addition to more formal medical treatment, not instead of it.

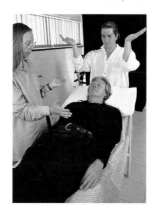

Healing occurs throughout the world and can occur by the "laying on of hands", or without physical touch from a distance.

Reiki

Reiki means "universal energy." Treatment by a Reiki practitioner promotes physical, emotional, and spiritual well-being. Healing is given when the practitioner's hands are placed on specific parts of the body, although some practitioners do not physically touch the body, but administer healing to the energy field (aura) surrounding the body. Reiki energies appear to provide a longer-lasting benefit when the recipients accept responsibility for the healing process.

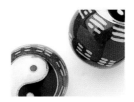

FENG SHUI
Feng shui is the art of maintaining harmony by achieving free movement of the universal life force, the Qi (see page 160). In their long practice of feng shui the Chinese have positioned their houses, furnishings, wells and even roads to be in harmony with the energy of the Earth. For them, correcting bad feng shui is essential for healing.

Self-help feng shui includes:
- Having plenty of plants and flowers both at home and work: some plants have the capacity to absorb some of the toxic chemicals found in modern buildings.

- Having a laundry basket to keep dirty clothes tidy before being washed, and doing any necessary mending as soon as it is needed; otherwise items are not put away.

- Throwing out old clothes and cosmetics, and out-of-date medicines and packets or cans of food.

- Tidying drawers.

- Sorting out personal papers and taking newspapers for recycling on a regular basis.

- Having a clean and tidy desk at work.

Geopathic therapy

Geopathic therapy aims to relieve any stress caused by the natural energy of the Earth. This energy form has been recognized for thousands of years, but was probably easier to detect before industrialization. Geopathic therapists believe that ancient cultures located their religious and other significant sites where the Earth's energy was particularly strong. Such sites may, in part, reflect the electromagnetic fields that can be associated with specific types of soil, and detected by trained dowsers. Dowsers are, in some way, sensitive to very small changes in electromagnetic fields, which appear to affect the way their muscles contract. This effect is transmitted to a pendulm or dowser's rod, held in the hand. Adverse energy can sometimes be avoided by moving a bed or chair. Alternatively, practitioners of geopathic therapy believe that negative energy can be deflected with mirrors, or captured in crystals or coils that can then be cleansed. Such treatment may help insomnia, headaches, digestive symptoms, anxiety, or depression.

FLOWER
REMEDIES
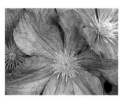
Today, in the West, the name that is probably most frequently associated with flower remedies is Dr. Edward Bach (pronounced batch). Practicing in London in the early twentieth century, he noticed that his patients' psychological responses to disease varied greatly and came to believe that emotional problems caused illness. He searched for a therapy that would reduce the negative emotional attitudes that he had observed in his patients, and found that flower essences were beneficial. Bach developed 38 remedies, but today additional flower remedies have been prepared from flowers that grow throughout the world.

Flower remedies are made in two ways. One method is to float freshly picked flowers in water, which is then left in full sunlight for three hours. The other method is to boil flowering twigs in water for half an hour. The resulting liquid is strained and a portion is diluted with an equal volume of brandy before being stored in a clean amber-colored glass bottle.

Crystal and gem therapy

Crystal and gem therapy is used by healers who believe that crystals have the power to focus and strengthen healing energies. An extension of this belief is the use of gems and crystals in various places around the house to absorb negative energy from geopathic stress (see box, page 179) or electrical pollution, especially from computer and television screens. Crystals used in this way should be washed regularly in cold running water and left in the sun to recharge. There is little hard scientific evidence to support the beneficial effects of using crystals in this way, but those who have used them believe that they can be helpful for stress and chronically painful conditions.

Rescue remedy

Rescue remedy is made from five of Bach's remedies: rock rose, impatiens, clematis, cherry plum, and star of Bethlehem. Put four drops in water and sip after an accident, argument, surgery, or any emotional, physical, or mental shock. Repeat as needed.

Using the flower remedies

The remedies are usually taken by sipping mineral water to which a few drops of the essence have been added. It is not certain how they work, although the action may be closer to homeopathy (see page 168) than to herbal medicines. Professional counselors and therapists often recommend them for use in addition to conventional medicines.

Conditions that can be treated with flower remedies include:

- Mood swings, including depression and anxiety.

- Nervous disorders, including lack of confidence, jealousy, and apathy.

- Sudden emotional, physical, or mental shock.

(This list is not intended to be comprehensive. Flower remedies are helpful for self-help as a first-aid treatment, but it is best to ask your doctor's advice about longer-term problems.)

Flower remedies can be made by floating freshly picked flowers in water and leaving them in the sun for three hours.

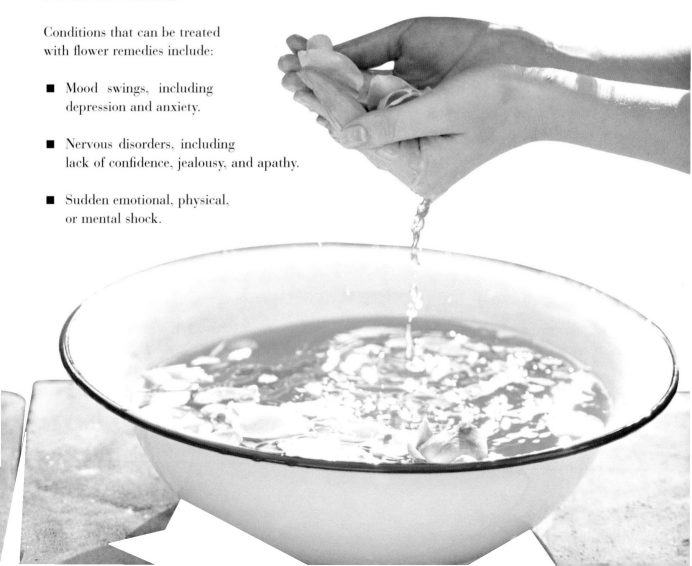

GUIDE TO CHOOSING **YOUR THERAPY**

Ideally, you should have your doctor's agreement before either consulting a practitioner of natural medicine or using any of these treatments as self-help remedies. This is because it is essential to have a diagnosis, and to be reassured that your symptoms are not the first symptoms of a serious disease that needs surgery or other conventional treatment. The list provided here offers some guidance as to which treatment may be helpful for certain conditions. It is not exhaustive because individuals vary greatly and symptoms can have more than one cause.

ADDICTIONS acupuncture, aromatherapy, counseling, hypnotherapy, massage, meditation, psychotherapy, yoga

ALLERGIES Alexander technique, fasting, herbal medicine, homeopathy, reflexology, relaxation therapies

ALZHEIMER'S DISEASE herbal medicine, homeopathy

ANGINA acupuncture, herbal medicine, homeopathy,

ANXIETY acupuncture, Alexander technique, aromatherapy, Bach flower remedies, counseling, herbal medicine, homeopathy, hydrotherapy, hypnotherapy, massage, meditation, nutrition therapy, relaxation, visualization, yoga

ARTHRITIS acupuncture, aromatherapy, balneotherapy, chiropractic, healing, herbal medicine, homeopathy, hydrotherapy, massage, nutrition therapy, osteopathy, peat therapy, yoga

ASTHMA acupressure, acupuncture, Alexander technique, Bach flower remedies, bioenergetics, chiropractic, homeopathy, hydrotherapy, meditation, nutrition therapy, osteopathy, reflexology, yoga

ATHLETE'S FOOT aromatherapy, herbal medicine

BACK PAIN acupressure, acupuncture, chiropractic, hydrotherapy, massage, osteopathy, reflexology

BEREAVEMENT *see* grief

CANKER SORES, COLD SORES, and GENITAL HERPES aromatherapy, herbal medicine, homeopathy, nutrition therapy

CARPAL TUNNEL SYNDROME acupressure, acupuncture, hydrotherapy, nutrition therapy, osteopathy

CATARACTS nutrition therapy

CHRONIC FATIGUE SYNDROME acupuncture, aromatherapy, counseling, herbal medicine, homeopathy, hypnotherapy, meditation, nutrition therapy, reflexology, relaxation, yoga

COLDS, COUGHS, THE FLU acupressure, acupuncture, aromatherapy, herbal medicine, homeopathy, naturopathy, nutrition therapy

CONSTIPATION acupuncture, herbal medicine, massage, nutrition therapy, reflexology

CYSTITIS acupressure, acupuncture, aromatherapy, herbal medicine, homeopathy, nutrition therapy

DEPRESSION aromatherapy, Bach flower remedies, cognitive therapy, color therapy, counseling, homeopathy, hypnotherapy, massage, psychotherapy, reflexology, yoga

DIARRHEA acupressure, herbal medicine, homeopathy, naturopathy, nutrition therapy

DIVERTICULITIS acupuncture, herbal medicine, massage, nutrition therapy, reflexology

ECZEMA/DERMATITIS acupuncture, aromatherapy, Chinese herbs, herbal medicine, homeopathy, hydrotherapy, nutrition therapy

EDEMA acupressure, aromatherapy, herbal medicine, massage

ERECTION PROBLEMS aromatherapy, herbal medicine, hydrotherapy

FAINTING acupressure, Bach flower remedies

FECAL INCONTINENCE acupressure, homeopathy, nutrition therapy, yoga

FIBROSITIS acupressure, acupuncture, biochemic tissue salts, chiropractic, healing, herbal medicine, homeopathy, hypnotherapy, massage, myotherapy, nutrition therapy, osteopathy, Rolfing, shiatsu

FROZEN SHOULDER acupressure, acupuncture, aromatherapy, chiropractic, herbal medicine, homeopathy, hydrotherapy, massage, osteopathy, TENS

GAS herbal medicine, nutrition therapy, reflexology

GASTROENTERITIS herbal medicine, homeopathy, nutrition therapy

GOUT acupressure, chiropractic, herbal medicine, homeopathy, massage, nutrition therapy, osteopathy

GRIEF counseling, homeopathy

HANGOVER homeopathy, naturopathy

HAY FEVER acupressure, aromatherapy, homeopathy, nutrition therapy

HEADACHES acupressure, chiropractic, herbal medicine, homeopathy, hydrotherapy, osteopathy

HEAT RASH aromatherapy, homeopathy, nutrition therapy

HEMORRHOIDS and VARICOSE VEINS aromatherapy, herbal medicine, homeopathy, hydrotherapy, nutrition therapy, yoga

HIGH BLOOD PRESSURE acupressure, acupuncture, aromatherapy, herbal medicine, homeopathy, hydrotherapy, hypnotherapy, nutrition therapy, yoga

INDIGESTION and HEARTBURN aromatherapy, herbal medicine, homeopathy, nutrition therapy, relaxation therapies

INSOMNIA Alexander technique, bioenergetics, homeopathy, hydrotherapy, massage, meditation

IRRITABLE BOWEL SYNDROME acupuncture, aromatherapy, counseling, fasting, herbal medicine, homeopathy, hypnotherapy, massage, meditation, nutrition therapy, yoga

JET LAG aromatherapy, herbal medicine, homeopathy

LIBIDO PROBLEMS aromatherapy, chi kung, counseling, Rolfing

ME (myalgic encephalomyelitis) *see* chronic fatigue syndrome

MENOPAUSE acupuncture, aromatherapy, herbal medicine, homeopathy, nutrition therapy

MENORRHAGIA (heavy periods) acupuncture, aromatherapy, homeopathy, nutrition therapy

MIGRAINES acupuncture, Alexander technique, aromatherapy, herbal medicine, homeopathy, massage, meditation, nutrition therapy, reflexology, relaxation therapies, shiatsu, yoga

NAUSEA acupressure, aromatherapy, nutrition therapy, herbal medicine, homeopathy, naturopathy

NEURALGIA acupressure, acupuncture, aromatherapy, homeopathy, hypnotherapy, naturopathy

OBESITY fasting, homeopathy, naturopathy, nutrition therapy

PAIN acupressure, acupuncture, Alexander technique, aromatherapy, chiropractic, healing, hydrotherapy, hypnotherapy, massage, meditation, nutrition therapy, osteopathy, psychotherapy, relaxation therapies, TENS

PHLEGM acupuncture, aromatherapy, herbal medicine, homeopathy, nutrition therapy

PROSTATE ENLARGEMENT acupuncture, herbal medicine, homeopathy

REPETITIVE STRAIN INJURY acupressure, acupuncture,

Alexander technique, chiropractic, homeopathy, hydrotherapy, massage, osteopathy

RESTLESS LEG SYNDROME acupuncture, herbal medicine, homeopathy, massage, nutrition therapy, osteopathy

SEASONAL AFFECTIVE DISORDER (SAD) aromatherapy, cognitive therapy, herbal medicine, light therapy, psychotherapy, relaxation therapies

SHINGLES acupuncture, aromatherapy, herbal medicine, homeopathy, nutrition therapy

SPRAINS acupuncture, aromatherapy, chiropractic, homeopathy, massage, osteopathy, TENS

STRESS aromatherapy, herbal medicine, homeopathy, hydrotherapy, massage, meditation, nutrition therapy, psychotherapy, reflexology, relaxation therapies, visualization, yoga

STROKE acupressure, biochemic tissue salts, chiropractic, herbal medicine, homeopathy, hydrotherapy, massage, nutrition therapy, osteopathy, yoga

SUNBURN aromatherapy, herbal medicine, homeopathy, hydrotherapy, naturopathy

TINNITUS osteopathy, reflexology, yoga

URINARY INCONTINENCE acupuncture, homeopathy, nutrition therapy

URTICARIA aromatherapy, herbal medicine, homeopathy

VARICOSE VEINS *see* hemorrhoids

WARTS aromatherapy, herbal medicine, homeopathy

WHIPLASH acupuncture, Alexander technique, aromatherapy, chiropractic, homeopathy, hydrotherapy, massage, osteopathy

USEFUL ADDRESSES

Acupuncture

Acupuncture Foundation of
Canada
2131 Lawrence Avenue East
Toronto
Ontario M1R 5G4
Canada
Tel: 1 416 752 3988
www.afcinstitute.com

National Acupuncture and
Oriental Medicine Alliance
(National Alliance)
14637 Starr Road
Olall, WA 98359
USA
Tel: 1 253 851 6896
Fax: 1 253 851 6883
www.acuall.org

Alexander Technique

American Society of the
Alexander Technique
401 East Market Street
Charlottesville, VA 2290
USA
Tel: 1 800 473 0620/ 1 804 295
2840
Fax: 1 804 295 3949
www.alexandertech.org
Email:alexanertec@earthlink.com

Canadian Society of Teachers of
the Alexander Technique
(CANSTAT)
465 Wilson Avenue
Toronto
Ontario M3H 1T9
Canada
Tel: 1 877 598 8879
www.canstat.ca

Aromatherapy

Canadian Federation of
Aromatherapists
868 Markham Road
Suite 109
Scarborough
Ontario M1H 2Y2
Canada
Tel: 1 416 439 4884
www.interlog.com/~aromaspa

Bach Flower Remedies

Nelson Back USA Ltd.
Wilmington Technology Park
100 Research Drive
Wilmington, MA 01887-4406
USA
Tel: 1 978 988 3833
Fax: 1 978 988 0233
www.nelsonback.com

Biofeedback

Association for Applied
Psychophysiology and
Biofeedback
10200 West 44th Avenue
Apt 304
Wheat Ridge, CO 80033-8436
USA
Tel: 1 303 422 8436
Fax: 1 303 422 8894
www.aapb.org

Chiropractic

American Chiropractic
Association
1701 Clarendon Boulevard
Arlington, VA 22209
USA
Tel: 1 703 276 8800
Fax: 1 703 243 2593
www.acatoday.com

Canadian Chiropractic
Association
1396 Eglington Avenue West
Toronto
Ontario M6C 2E4
Canada
Tel: 1 416 781 5656
Fax: 1 416 781 7344
www.ccachiro.org

Counseling

American Counciling
Association
5999 Stevenson Avenue
Alexandria, VA 22304-3300
USA
Tel: 1 703 823 9800
Fax: 1 703 823 0252
www.counceling.org

Dreamwork

Association for the Study of
Dreams
6728 Old McLean Village Drive
McLean, VA 22101
USA
Tel: 1 703 556 0739
Fax: 1 703 556 8729
www.asdreams.org

Expression Therapies

American Art Therapy
Association
1202 Allanson Road
Mundelein, Il 60060
USA
Tel: 1 847 949 6064
Fax: 1 847 566 4580
www.arttherapy.org

American Dance Therapy
Association
2000 Century Plaza, Suite 108
Columbia, MA 21044
USA
Tel: 1 410 997 4040
Fax: 1 410 997 4048
www.adta.org

Laban/Bartenieff Institute of
Movement Studies
234 Fifth Avenue, Room 203
New York, NY 10001
USA
Tel: 1 212 477 4299
Fax: 1 212 477 3702
www.limsonline.org

National Association of Music
Therapy
8455 Colesville Road
Suite 1000
Silver Spring, Maryland 20910
USA
Tel: 1 301 589 3300
Fax: 1 301 589 5175
www.musictherapy.org

Gestalt Therapy

Gestalt Center for Psychotherapy
and Training
26 West 9th Street

New York, NY
USA
Tel: 1 212 387 9429

Gestalt Therapy Institute of the
Pacific
Faculty Training Office
1626 Westwood Boulevard
Suite 104
Los Angeles, CA 90024
USA
Tel: 1 310 446 9720
Fax: 1 310 475 4704
www.gestalttherapy.org.uk
email:Lynnejacobs@bigfoot.com
OR gyontef@gestalt.org

Hellerwork

Hellerwork International
406 Berry Street
Mount Shasta, CA 96067
USA
Tel: 1 707 441 4949
Fax: 1 530 926 5839
www.hellerwork.com

Holistic Medicine

American Holistic Health
Association
PO Box 17400
Anaheim, CA 92817-7400
USA
Tel: 1 714779 6152
www.ahha.org

American Holistic Medical
Association
6728 Old McLean Village Drive
McLean, VA 22101
USA
Tel: 1 703 556 9728
Fax: 1 703 556 8729
www.holisticmedicine.org
email: kitty@degnon.org

Homeopathy

Homeopathic Educational
Services
2124 Kittredge St
Berkeley, CA 94704
USA
Tel: 1 510 649 0294
Fax: 1 510 649 1955
www.homeopathic.com
Email: mail@homeopathic.com

Homeopathic Council for
Research and Education
50 Park Avenue East
New York, NY 10016
USA
Tel: 1 212 864 2290
Fax: 1 212 684 4694

National Center for
Homeopathy
801 North Fairfax Street
Suite 306
Alexandria, VA 22314
USA
Tel: 1 703 548 7790
Fax: 1 703 548 7792
www.homeopathic.org

Massage

American Massage Therapy
Association
820 Davis Street
Suite 100
Evanston, Ill 60201-4444
USA
Tel: 1 847 864 0123
Fax: 1 847 864 1178
www.amtamassage.org

Associated Bodywork and
Massage Professionals
1271 Sugar Bush Drive
Evergreen, CO 80439
USA
Tel: 1 303 674 8478
Fax: 1 303 674 0859
www.abmp.com

Canadian Massage Therapists
Alliance
365 Bloor Street East
Suite 1807
Toronto
Ontario M4W 3L4
Canada
Tel: 1 416 968 2149
www.collinscan.com/~collins/
clientspgs/cmtai.html

International Massage
Association
92 Main Street
PO Drawer 421
Warrenton, VA 20188-0421
USA
Tel: 1 540 351 0800
Fax: 1540 351 0816
www.imagroup.com

Skilled Touch Institute of Chair
Massage
584 Castro Street
Suite 555
San Francisco, CA 94114-2588
USA
Tel: 1 415 861 4746
Fax: 1 415 621 1260
www.touchpro.org

Naturopathy

American Association of
Naturopathic Physicians
601 Valley Street
Seattle, WA 98102
USA
Tel: 1 206 298 0125
www.naturopathic.org

American Naturopathic Medical
Association
PO Box 96273
Las Vegas, NV 89193
USA
Tel: 1 702 897 7053
www.anma.com

Canadian Naturopathic
Association
1255 Sheppard Avenue
East
North York
Ontario M2K 1E2
Canada
Tel: 1 416 496 8633
www.naturopathicassoc.ca

Nutrition and Diet Therapy

American Dietetics
Association
216 West Jackson Boulevard
Apt 800
Chicago, Ill 60606-6995
USA
Tel: 1 800 877 1600
Fax: 1 212 899 4758
www.eatright.org

National Institute of Nutrition
265 Carling Avenue
Suite 302
Ottawa
Ontario K1S 2E1
Tel: 1 613 235 3355
http://www.nin.ca

Oriental Medicine

American Association of Oriental
Medicine (AAOM)
433 Front Street
Catasauqua, PA 18032
USA
Tel: 1 610 266 1433
Fax: 1 610 264 2768
www.aaom.org

James MacRitchie and Damaris
Jarboux
Chi Kung School at the Body-
Energy Center
PO Box 19708
Boulder, CO 80308
USA
Tel: 1 303 442 3131
Fax: 1 303 442 3141
email:jamesmacritchie@earth-
link.net

Qigong Academy
5553 Pearl Road
Cleveland, OH 44129
USA
Tel/Fax: 1 440 842 8042
www.qigongacademy.com

Osteopathy

American Academy of
Osteopathy
3500 DePauw Boulevard
Suite 1080
Indianapolis, IN 46268-139
USA
Tel: 1 317 879 1881
Fax: 1 317 879 0563
www.academyofosteopathy.
org

American Osteopathic
Association
142 East Ontario Street
Chicago, Il 60611
USA
Tel: 1 312 202 8000
Fax: 1 312 202 8200
www.aoa-net.org

Canadian Osteopathic
Association
575 Waterloo Street
London
Ontario N6B 2R2
Tel: 1 519 439 5521

Polarity Therapy

American Polarity Therapy
Association
PO Box 19858
Boulder, CO 80308
USA
Tel: 1 303 545 2080
Fax: 1 303 545 2161
www.polaritytherapy.org

Zero Balancing Associaton
PO Box 1727
Capitola, CA 95010
USA
Tel: 1 831 476 0665
Fax: 1 831 475 0525

Reflexology

Association of Vacuflex
Reflexology
718 Arnold Avenue
Point Pleasant, NJ 08742
USA
Tel: 1 732 892 7566
Fax: 1 732 892 0947

Reflexology Association of
Canada
Unit 1B
5000 Dufferin Street
Toronto
Ontario M3H 5T5
Tel: 1 416 663 2114
www.reflexologycanada.ca

Reiki

Center for Reiki Traning
21421 Hilltop St 28
Southfield
MI 48034
USA
Tel: 1 248 948 8112
Fax: 1 248 948 9534
www.reiki.org

Rolfing

The Rolf Institute
205 Canyon Boulevard
Boulder, CO 80302-4920
USA
Tel: 1 303 449 5903
Fax: 1 303 449 5978
www.rolf.org

Shamanism

Cross-Cultural Shamanism
Network
PO Box 270
William, OR 97504
USA
Tel: 1 541 846 1313
Fax: 1 541 846 1204

Foundation for Shamanic
Studies
PO Box 1939
Mill Valley, CA 94942
USA
Tel: 1 415 380 8282
Fax: 1 415 380 8416
www.shamanism.org

Yoga

BKS Iyengar Yoga National
Association of the US
8223 West 3rd Street
Los Angeles, CA 90088
USA
Tel: 1 323 653 0357

International Association of Yoga
Therapists (a division of The
Yoga Research and Education
Centre)
PO Box 1386
Lower Lake, CA 95457
USA
Tel: 1 707 928 9898
Fax: 1 707 928 4738
www.yrec.org

Sivananda Yoga Vedanta Centre
243 West 24th Street
New York, NY 10011
USA
Tel: 1 212 255 4560
Fax: 1 212 727 7392
www.sivananda.org

Sivananda Yoga Vedanta Centre
5178 St Lawrence Boulevard
Montreal
Quebec H2T 1R8
Canada
Tel: 1 514 279 3545
Fax: 1 514 279 3527
email: montreal@sivananda.org

BIBLIOGRAPHY

Part 1

Aphrodite Diet, The
Simopoulos, Artemis, P. and
Robinson, J.
Vermillion, London, UK, 1999

Book of Pain Relief, The
Chaitow, L.
Thorsons, London, UK, 1993

Complete Book of Walking, The
Kuntzlemann, C. T.
Simon and Schuster, New York,
US, 1978

*Dietary Reference Values for
Food and Energy and Nutrients
for the United Kingdom*
The Stationery Office, London,
UK, 1991

Exercise Beats Arthritis
Sayce, V. and Fraser, I.
Thorsons, 2nd edition, London,
UK, 1992

Fats That Heal, Fats That Kill
Erasmus, U.
Alive Books, 1993

Getting Older Slowly
Franks, H.
Rosendale Press Ltd, London,
UK, 1994

Longevity Strategy, The
Mahoney, D. and Restak, R.
John Wiley and Sons, Inc., New
York, US, 1998

*Nutritional Aspects of the
Development of Cancer*
The Stationery Office, London,
UK, 1998

*Osteoporosis Prevention
Guide, The*
Brewer, Dr S.
Souvenir Press, London, UK,
1998

*Recommended Daily Allowances
10th edition*
National Academy Press,
Washington, US

Staying Healthy with Nutrition
Haas, E., MD
Celestial Arts, UK, 1992

Vitamin Alphabet, The
Scott-Moncrieff, Dr C. M.
Collins & Brown, London, UK,
1999

Part 2

Acupressure
Young, J.
Thorsons, London, UK, 1994

Acupuncture
Hicks, A.
Thorsons, London, UK, 1997

*Anxiety, Phobias and Panic
Attacks*
Sheehan, E.
Element Books, Shaftesbury,
UK, 1996

Aromatherapy
Wildwood, C.
Bloomsbury Publishing,
London, UK, 1996

Book of Pain Relief, The
Chaitow, L.
Thorsons, London, UK, 1993

*Complete Family Guide to
Alternative Medicine, The*
Shealy, N. C. (Consultant Ed.)
Element, Shaftesbury, UK, 1996

Complete Medicinal Herbal
Ody, P.
Dorling Kindersley, London, UK,
1993

Family Guide to Reflexology, The
Gillanders, A.
Gaia Books Ltd, London, UK,
1998

Natural Therapies
Evans, M.
Select Editions, 1999

Pilates: The Way Forward
Robinson, L. and Thomson, G.
Pan Books, London, UK, 1999

Principles of Psychotherapy
Avery, B.
Thorsons, London, UK, 1996

Textbook of Natural Medicine
Pizzorno Jr. J. E. and Murray, M.
T. (Eds)
Churchill Livingstone, 2nd
edition, London, UK, 1999

Yoga for Common Ailments
Nagarathna, R., Nagendra, H. R.
and Monro, R.
Gaia Books Ltd, London, UK,
1990

INDEX

ACKNOWLEDGMENTS

Photographs copyright © as follows:

Page 2–3 Bob Thomas/Gettyone Stone: page 6 (knockback and inset) The Stock Market Photo Agency: page 8(tl) BSIP, Chassenet/Science Photo Library: page 8 (bl) The Stock Market Photo Agency: page 9 Bruce Ayres/Gettyone Stone: page 10 Lori Adamski Peek/Gettyone Stone: page 12 Laurence Monneret/Gettyone Stone: page 14 (knockback) Lori Adamski Peek/Gettyone Stone: page 16 (tl) BSIP, Taulin/Science Photo Library: page 21 BSIP, Chassenet/Science Photo Library: page 29 Lori Adamski Peek/Gettyone Stone: page 31 Richard Open/Camera Press: page 32 BSIP, Chassenet/Science Photo Library: page 34 (t) Bob Thomas/Gettyone Stone: page 34 (b) Al Franevich/The Stock Market Photo Agency: page 36 (t) BSIP, Chassenet/Science Photo Library: page 36 (b) The Stock Market Photo Agency: page 36 (knockback) BSIP, Zarand/Science Photo Library: page 38 (b) The Stock Market Photo Agency: page 39 Klaus Lahnstein/Gettyone Stone: page 40 (t) Steve Read/Gettyone Stone: page 40 (b) Sue Ford/Science Photo Library: page 41 Jane Shemilt/Science Photo Library: page 42 (cl) Martin Dohrn/Science Photo Library: page 43 The Stock Market Photo Agency: page 45 Science Photo Library: page 46 (b) M.Keller/The Stock Market Photo Agency: page 50 Walter Hodges/Gettyone Stone: page 51 The Stock Market Photo Agency: page 52 (top and knockback) The Stock Market Photo Agency: page 54 (t) Lori Adamski Peek/Gettyone Stone: page 54 (b) Aaron Strong/Gettyone Stone: page 55 (b) Ian O'Leary/Gettyone Stone: page 56 (b) Raota/Camera Press: page 57 The Stock Market Photo Agency: page 58 (t) Candice Farmer/Telegraph Colour Library: page 58 (b) Stuart McClymont/Gettyone Stone: page 59 (t) Walter Hodges/Gettyone Stone: page 59 (b) The Stock Market Photo Agency: page 60 (b) The Stock Market Photo Agency: page 61 (inset and knockbacked) The Stock Market Photo Agency: page 62 (top and bottom) The Stock Market Photo Agency: page 64 Barton/The Stock Maret Photo Agency: page 65 Bob Thomas/Gettyone Stone: page 66 (t and br) BSIP, Vem/Science Photo Library: page 66 (bl) NIBSC/Science Photo Library: page 68 David Madison/Gettyone Stone: page 69 Jane Hancer/Camera Press: page 70 (t) Jane Shemilt/Science Photo Library: page 70 (knockback) Adam Hart-Davis/Science Photo Library: page 71 The Stock Market Photo Agency: page 72 Bob Thomas/Gettyone Stone: page 73 (t) The Stock Market Photo Agency: page 73 (b) CNRI/Science Photo Library: page 74 (b) James Stevenson/Science Photo Library: page 75 The Stock Market Photo Agency: page 76 (t) Biophoto Associates/Science Photo Library: page 76 (knockback) BSIP, Alexandre/Science Photo Library: page 77 M.Keller/The Stock Market Photo Agency: page 80 (t) The Stock Market Photo Agency: page 80 (b) T. Wood/Camera Press: page 80 (knockback) Leonardo Cendamo Ag. Grazia Neri/Camera Press: page 81 Gisela Them/Camera Press: page 83 (top and bottom) The Stock Market Photo Agency: page 84 (t) The Stock Market Photo Agency: page 85 Axel Springer Verlag Ag/Camera Press: page 86 The Stock Market Photo Agency: page 87 Martin Barraud/Gettyone Stone: page 88 (t) Amwell/Gettyone Stone: page 88 (b) Lori Adamski Peek/Gettyone Stone: page 89 Ron Chapple/Telegraph Colour Library: page 90 (t) The Stock Market Photo Agency: page 90 (b) Jim Cummins/Telegraph Colour Library: page 91 Dr. M.Goedert/Science Photo Library: page 92 (t) The Stock Market Photo Agency: page 92 (b) Ron Chapple/Telegraph Colour Library: page 93 The Stock Market Photo Agency: page 94 Axel Springer Verlag Ag/Camera Press: page 95 The Stock Market Photo Agency: page 98 M.Keller/The Stock Market Photo Agency: page 99 Quelle/Them/Camera Press: page 100 (top and bottom) The Stock Market Photo Agency: page 101 Sue Dent/ Hutchison Library: page 102 Fair Lady/Camera Press: page 103 (b) Faye Norman/Science Photo Library: page 103 (t) Amwell/Gettyone Stone: page 104 Candice Farmer/Telegraph Colour Library: page 105 D.Luria/Telegraph Colour Library: page 106 Steve Reed/Gettyone Stone: page 108 (t) Stewart Cohen/Gettyone Stone: page 108 (b) Dankloff/Camera Press: page 109 Martin Barraud/ Gettyone Stone: page 110 The Stock Market Photo Agency: page 113 The Stock Market Photo Agency: page 114 (t) Rush/Camera Press: page 114 (b) The Stock Market Photo Agency: page 116 The Stock Market Photo Agency: page 119 Tony Souter/Hutchison Library: page 120 (b) Axel Springer Verlag Ag/Camera Press: page 122 Camera Press: page 124–125 James Darell/Gettyone Stone: page 126 Bob Thomas/Gettyone Stone: page 129 Bob Thomas/Gettyone Stone: page 138 The Stock Market Photo Agency: page 140 (b) Nick Haslam/Hutchison Library: page 141 Rush/Camera Press: page 143 (t) Jerrican Agency/Power Stock Photo Library: page 145 Eva Vermandel/Time Out/Camera Press: page 146 The Stock Market Photo Agency: page 147 The Stock Market Photo Agency: page 148 Eva Vermandel/Time Out/Camera Press: page 151 (t) Womens Value/ Camera Press: page 151 (b) Richard Open/Camera Press: page 153 Living Liv 642/Camera Press: page 160 Ali Russell/Camera Press: page 161 (bl) Axel Springer Verlag Ag/Camera Press: page 161 (br) Ali Russell/Camera Press: page 162 Richard Open/Camera Press: page 163 Camera Press: page 164 Richard Open/Camera Press: page 165 Tullio/Camera Press: page 166 Jacky Chapman/Format Photographers: page 167 IMS/Camera Press: page 168 Sue Dent/ Hutchison Library: page 169 IMA Press: Gilles Rolle/Camera Press: page 170 Stewart Cohen/Gettyone Stone: page 172 (knockback, top and bottom) Shaz/Camera Press: page 174 Ali Russell/Camera Press: page 175 Richard Open/Camera Press: page 176 David Raffan/Camera Press: page 177 David Raffan/Camera Press: page 178 (b) You/Camera Press: page 181 Picture Bank

Jacket, front: top left Laurence Monneret/Gettyone Stone: bottom left Aaron Strong/Gettyone Stone: bottom right Richard Open/Camera Press. Jacket, back: top right Ian O'Leary/Gettyone Stone: bottom left Ali Russell/Camera Press

All other photographs copyright © Collins and Brown